W9-AYI-142

The PORTABLE ESSENTIAL OILS

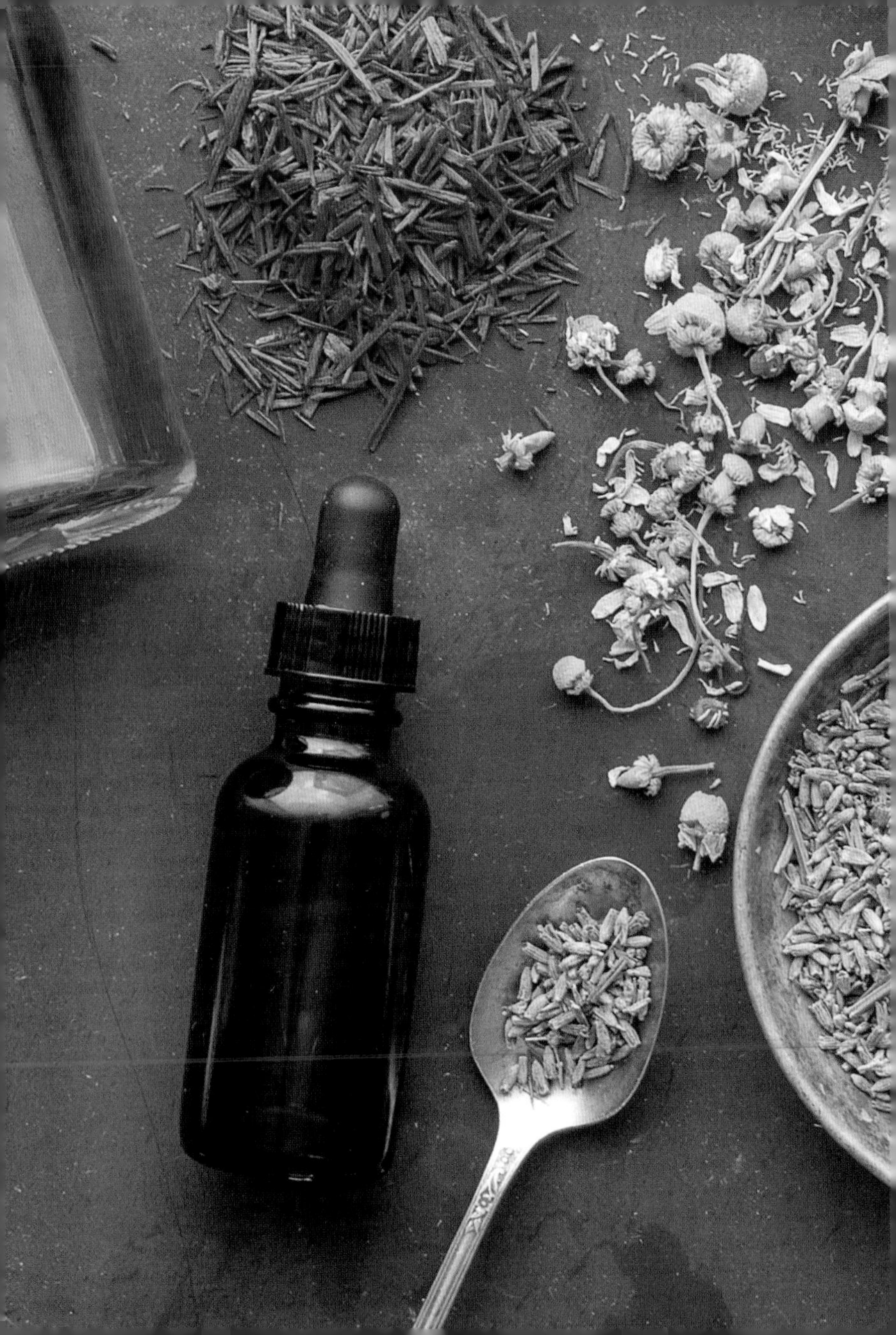

The PORTABLE ESSENTIAL OILS

A Pocket Reference *of* Everyday Remedies *for* Natural Health & Wellness

ANNE KENNEDY

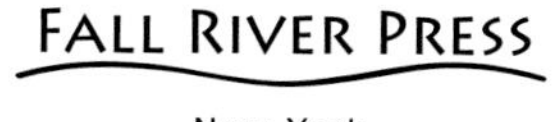

New York

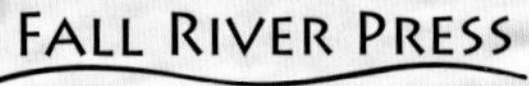

New York

An Imprint of Sterling Publishing Co., Inc.
1166 Avenue of the Americas
New York, NY 10036

FALL RIVER PRESS and the distinctive Fall River Press logo are registered trademarks of Barnes & Noble Booksellers, Inc.

This publication includes alternative therapies and is intended for informational purposes only. The publisher does not claim that this publication shall provide or guarantee any benefits, healing, cure, or any results in any respect. This publication is not intended to provide or replace conventional medical advice, treatment, or diagnosis or be a substitute to consulting with a physician or other licensed medical or health-care provider. The publisher shall not be liable or responsible in any respect for any use or application of any content contained in this publication or any adverse effects, consequence, loss, or damage of any type resulting or arising from, directly or indirectly, the use or application of any content contained in this publication. Any trademarks are the property of their respective owners, are used for editorial purposes only, and the publisher makes no claim of ownership and shall acquire no right, title, or interest in such trademarks by virtue of this publication.

ISBN 978-1-4351-6644-8

For information about custom editions, special sales, and premium and corporate purchases, please contact Sterling Special Sales at 800-805-5489 or specialsales@sterlingpublishing.com.

Manufactured in China

2 4 6 8 10 9 7 5 3 1

sterlingpublishing.com

Cover design by David Ter-Avanesyan

Interior photography © Shannon Douglas, p.2; Pixel Stories/Stocksy, p.5; Borislav Zhuykov/Stocksy, p.12 & 44; all others Shutterstock, iStock, Thinkstock & Dreamtime

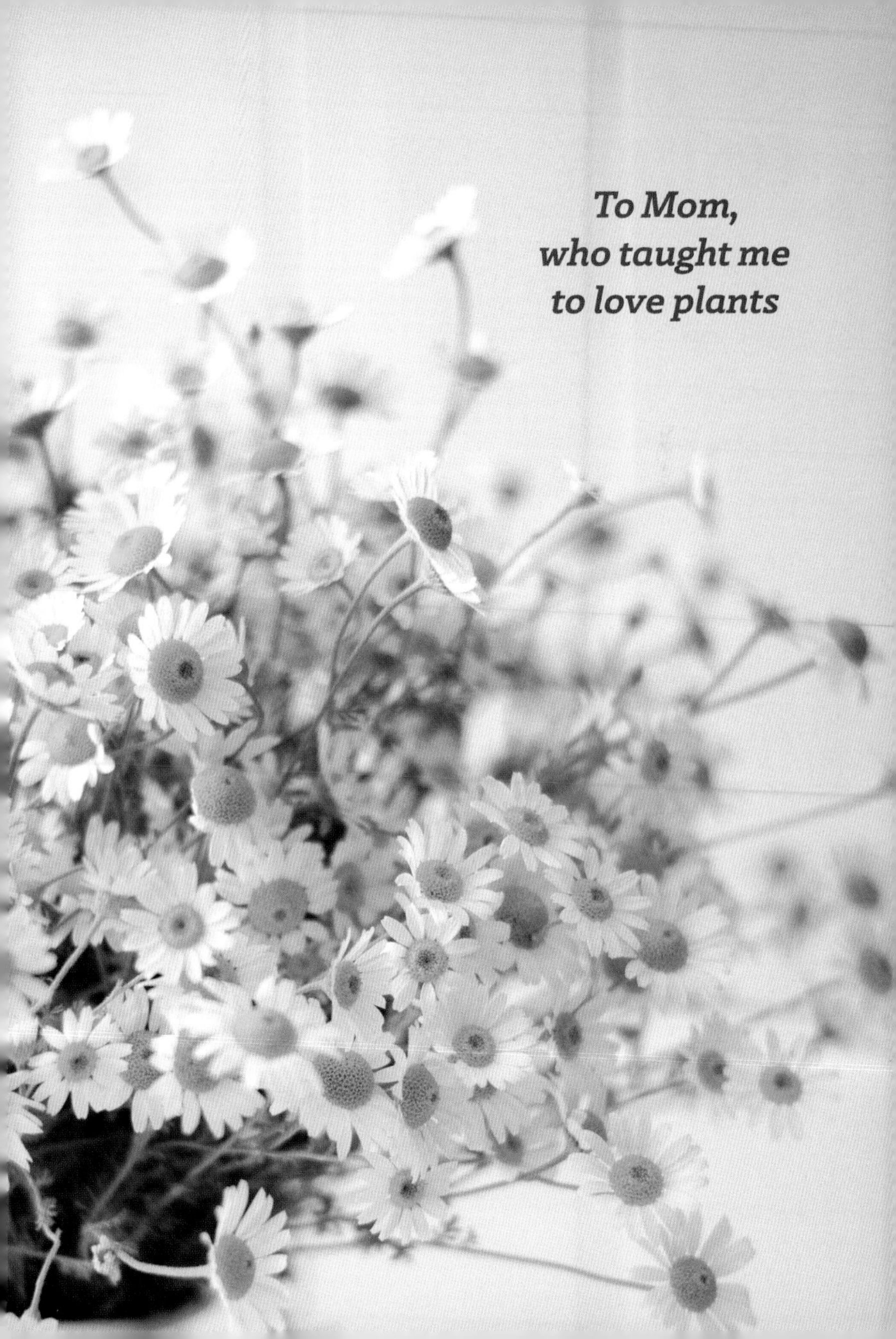

To Mom,
who taught me
to love plants

CONTENTS

PART THREE

50 Essential Oils in Profile

INTRODUCTION

Several months ago I traveled to a family reunion, opting to skip the hustle of air travel and enjoy a cross-country road trip. On the first night of my adventure, I found myself completely drained; even so, unfamiliar sounds and an uncomfortable bed kept me up. I rummaged through my bag, hoping to locate my lavender essential oil.

You guessed it—my favorite insomnia remedy was nowhere to be found, and I seriously doubted that the nearby convenience store could provide a replacement. The next day, bleary-eyed and chugging coffee, I searched frantically for a place to buy essential oils to get me through the rest of my trip.

Once I got my hands on a few versatile oils—lavender, peppermint, rosemary, and grapefruit—stress, insomnia, fatigue, and stuffy rooms had nothing on me. Inside a small handful of bottles, I had everything I needed to stay focused while driving across long stretches of empty highway, along with quick remedies for everything from the discomfort of fast food–induced indigestion to the annoyance of construction delays. With no pills to take and no side effects to worry about, plus pleasant aromas that kept me in a positive frame of mind, I enjoyed my long drive to the reunion.

Thanks to their wonderful healing powers and portability, essential oils now have a permanent place on my packing list. In fact, I have a little bottle of lavender that never leaves my purse. I have dozens of uses for it, and once you become familiar with the remedies in this take-anywhere guide, so will you. By preparing again and again the essential oil remedies described in this book, you'll be able to care for yourself and your family naturally, wherever you are.

The Portable Essential Oils is a handy guide that has you covered at any time, any place. Whether you're dealing with a tired, cranky kiddo while finishing up your Friday afternoon errands, or facing the potential for sunburn, mosquito bites, and poison ivy during a weekend camping trip, you'll find quick, simple remedies inside.

Part 1 offers safe, easy ways to put health and healing into your own hands, no medical training required. In Part 2, you'll find a list of A-to-Z ailments and corresponding remedies. Part 3 is where you'll learn more about the specific essential oils you can use individually or in the blends described. I've included profiles of 50 of the most versatile and largely inexpensive essential oils available. At the end of the book, you'll find a glossary, a handy ailments and oils quick-reference guide, and a quick guide to some top essential oil brands.

With a handful of essential oils and the information in this guide, you'll be prepared for just about anything.

PART ONE

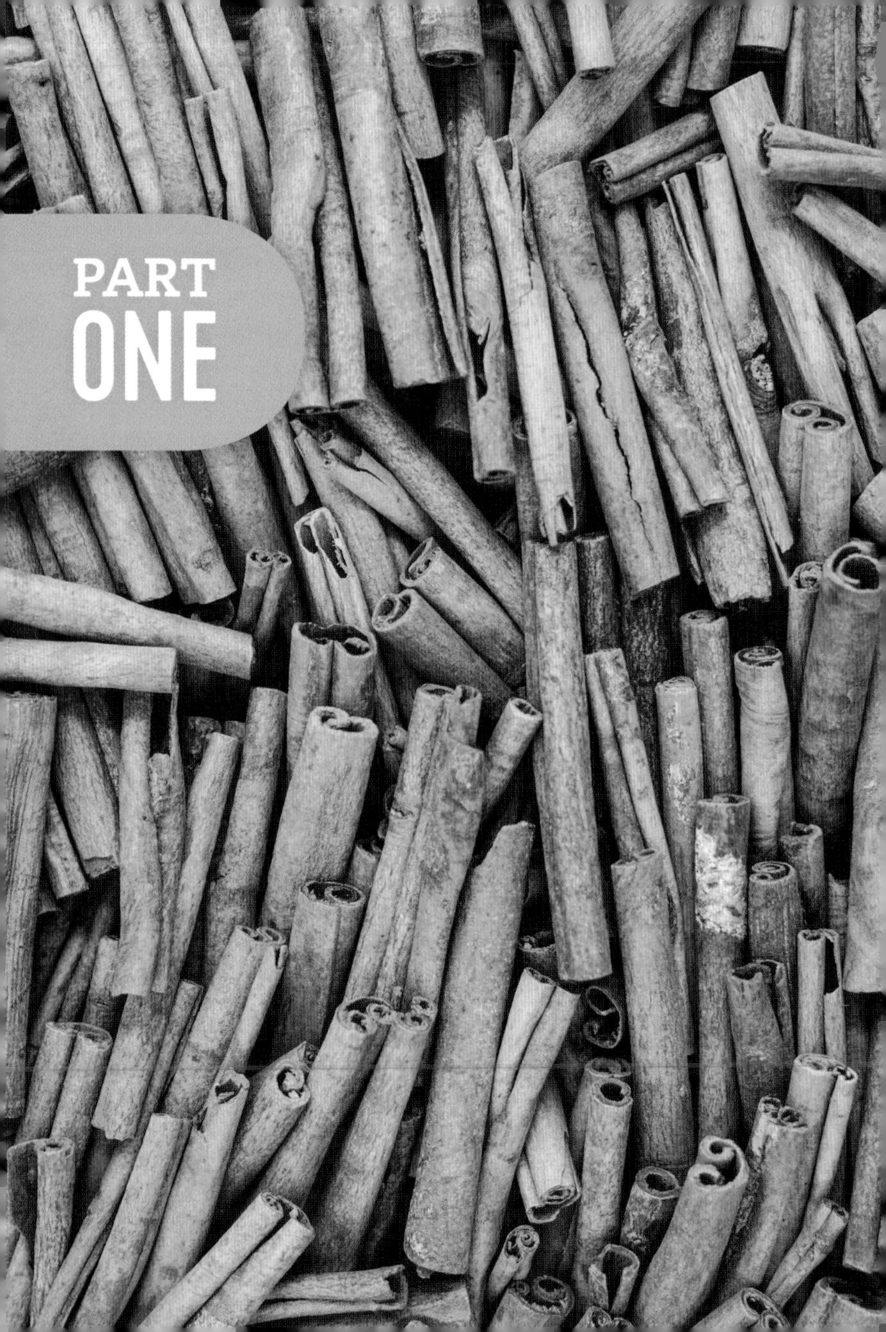

Health & Healing in Your Hands

Run a quick online search for essential oils, and you'll find a surprising amount of information, along with plenty of products vying for your attention. Look past the advertising and dig just a little deeper, and you'll discover that people from a variety of backgrounds use these powerful plant extracts to treat everything from asthma to yeast infections, and almost everything in between.

The explosion of essential oils interest and usage in recent years hasn't happened by mistake. People want to care for themselves and their families without worrying about scary side effects, and as most essential oils are safe, effective, and affordable, they often make good stand-ins for over-the-counter (OTC) medications. Once popular among just a few groups of people—including well-informed massage therapists and patchouli-scented hippies—essential oils are now readily available to anyone with an interest in natural health and healing.

If you're already familiar with essential oils, you probably know that they are not one-size-fits-all remedies. If you're brand new to the concept of treating common ailments with aromatic oils distilled from plants, you might feel a little intimidated. After all, there are more than 300 essential oils, and many of these come from exotic plants and trees you may have never heard of. Some even come from poisonous plant species, but don't worry: none of those are recommended here.

Where to begin? Whether you have been using essential oils for years or have been newly gifted with this friendly guide, knowing which essential oils to use for which ailments can seem like a bit of a guessing game. Conflicting online information doesn't help and can lead to confusion.

This section offers a concise, need-to-know overview that will help you make well-informed shopping decisions wherever you are, whenever you need to. You'll learn about the science of essential oils while gaining an awareness of the many benefits they provide. Additionally, you'll find tips that make shopping for oils easier, with insight into marketing claims, what to question, what to avoid, and how to read the labels.

Using the information you'll find here as a guide, you can also create a shopping list for simple tools and supplies you'll need for making, storing, and dispensing remedies. What's more, the important safety information and instructions for common aromatic and topical applications provided here should help you avoid common mistakes so that you can enjoy using essential oils with confidence.

SCENTS WITH INTENT

An uplifting scent can transform your mood in an instant. Just smelling fresh citrus can send stress into a downward spiral, and a sudden whiff of spice may evoke happy memories of holiday baking in Grandma's kitchen. In contrast, an overpowering or unpleasant aroma can do the opposite, making you look for a quick escape route.

Scents are powerful; they create immediate, visceral reactions in the body and mind. This includes their ability to bring about physical changes, such as healing, as well as changes to our emotions and moods.

Take peppermint, for example. Its sharp, fresh aroma has a positive effect on blood pressure, and it promotes the relaxation of bronchial smooth muscles, increasing breathing efficiency and increasing the amount of oxygen the bloodstream delivers to the brain. Inhaling peppermint to improve mental focus or enhance athletic performance is an illustration of aromatherapy in action. You'll gain insight into many other ways to use scents with intent as you read on.

What Is Aromatherapy?

When some people think of aromatherapy, colorful bottles of scented bath oil or body wash, or perhaps fragrant air fresheners in metal spray cans, come to mind. They might even think of perfumes, candles, or other fragranced products that mimic certain aromatic scents, thinking that if a desired fragrance is present, the product must offer the benefits of aromatherapy.

Unfortunately, many aromatherapy claims are marketing ploys. In actuality, aromatherapy is the intentional use of certain beneficial oils extracted from plants to enhance physical and/or psychological well-being. The molecular structures of essential oils are incredibly complex, giving plants the power to repel insects, recover from damage, resist viruses and bacteria, and more. Many of these plant extracts are the source of some of the same constituents found in modern medicines and antiseptics, making them so much more than fragrances alone.

A core component of aromatherapy, essential oils should not be confused with fragrance oils or perfumes. Pure essential oils contain no additives, whereas fragrance oils are heavily adulterated with chemicals that mimic scents found in nature. Because synthetic fragrance oils lack the potency of essential oils and may actually have a detrimental effect, they have no place in aromatherapy.

Aromatherapy really is scent with intent. Each essential oil has a distinct fragrance, and each offers specific properties that allow you to put it to practical use. Think of the wonderful fragrances as added benefits, and you'll understand that aromatherapy is all about health and healing.

BENEFITS OF ESSENTIAL OILS

Perhaps you have already experienced the healing benefits of essential oils, or maybe you have a few friends who swear by them. Physical healing is just one powerful reason to use essential oils. Here's more on that, plus other compelling reasons to add these all-natural extracts to your wellness regimen. Whether you want safe alternatives to OTC pain medications and sleep aids or are looking for easy ways to deal with common illnesses while saving some of your hard-earned dollars, essential oils can prove quite useful.

Health and Wellness

Just like some of the products found in pharmacies and on drugstore shelves, essential oils can help you feel better. For instance:

- Oils with *analgesic* properties ease pain.
- Oils with *antiseptic* properties help prevent infections by inhibiting the growth of dangerous microbes.
- Oils with *anti-inflammatory* properties help prevent and treat discomfort caused by inflammation and swelling.

These are just a few examples of the health benefits essential oils provide. As you read on, you'll discover that all 50 oils recommended in this book have numerous beneficial properties—for example, eucalyptus oil has analgesic, antiseptic, antiviral, and other benefits.

A Natural Alternative

Pure, unadulterated essential oils come straight from nature. They contain no waxes, dyes, fillers, or chemicals from questionable sources. When used correctly, they don't cause harmful side effects like those caused by common drugs. Using eucalyptus, peppermint, and lavender to deal with cold symptoms brings quick relief, and without the dry mouth, mental fog, and other undesirable effects some drugstore remedies bring with them. Medication residue can be tough on your body, particularly your liver. In contrast, essential oils are easy for your body to use, and they are completely expelled from your system in just a few hours.

Self-Empowered Healing

Essential oils allow you to assume greater responsibility for your health and improve your quality of life. Freedom from discomfort, deeper sleep, and the ability to handle difficulties such as stress and anxiety are some of the benefits you'll experience when you use essential oils to enhance your well-being. Vibrant energy and a positive mental outlook are additional benefits that go hand in hand with aromatherapy. By broadening your horizons and replacing chemical-based medicines with natural ones, you cut the pharmaceutical middleman from the equation. Over time, you'll gain the confidence to treat common illnesses without relying on others.

Lower Medical Bills

While it's not advisable to ditch your doctor, having the ability to use essential oils will help you and your family cut back on the number of conventional medical treatments you invest in each year. Knowing which essential oils to use for natural pain relief, which to use for migraines, and which to use for allergies, hay fever, earaches, and other common maladies can help you save money for other things. Treating problems like nail fungus, athlete's foot, and minor sprains on your own will lower your medical bills even more.

A BRIEF HISTORY OF ESSENTIAL OILS

Aromatic oils such as frankincense, sandalwood, and myrrh were popular with ancient Egyptians as long ago as 4500 BC. About 1,500 years later, Indian scholars developed Ayurveda, a system of natural healing still used today that incorporates essential oils into its treatments. Chinese doctors recorded the medicinal use of essential oils thousands of years ago, and the ancient Greeks and Romans used them, too. Numerous references to essential oils even appear throughout the Bible.

Stepping forward to the twentieth century, we find ourselves in the laboratory of French chemist René-Maurice Gattefossé, who sustained a major burn to his hand in a laboratory explosion. After submerging the injury in a vat of pure lavender essential oil, he was amazed to discover that he felt little pain and that he healed without infection or scarring. Later, Parisian doctor Jean Valnet ran out of antibiotics during a World War II shortage. He used essential oils to treat wounded soldiers and was surprised when the oils were able to reduce and even halt infections.

Today, with studies ongoing, essential oils are used in a wide range of settings around the world, including hospitals, to relieve pain, promote relaxation, improve mood, and more.

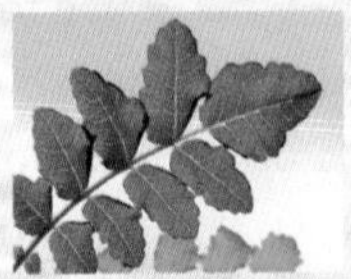

Frankincense

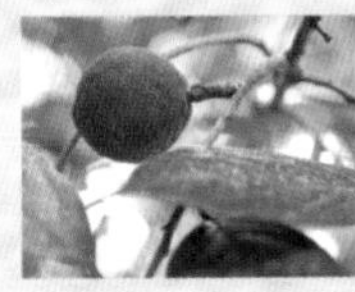

Sandalwood

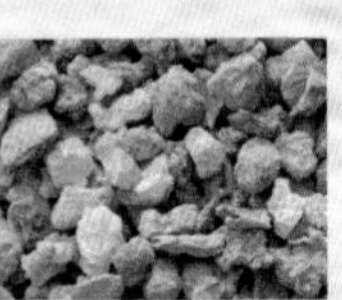

Myrrh

SCIENCE OF ESSENTIAL OILS

While the body of scientific research being conducted on essential oil effectiveness is still growing, there's no disputing the healing properties of plants. Many contain compounds that fight harmful bacteria, viruses, and fungi, and still others contain constituents that ease pain, ward off inflammation, diminish depression, and perform a variety of other useful functions.

Essential oils and the plants from which they are derived have long been used in pharmaceuticals and body-care products. Even modern drugs contain active ingredients derived from plants, or they use chemical copies of those constituents.

Essential oils are made up of tiny molecules that easily penetrate the skin, lungs, and other body systems, quickly making their way into the bloodstream. For instance:

- When you add a few drops of lavender oil to a bedtime bath, its molecules are absorbed two ways: Steam from the hot water delivers them to your respiratory system, and your skin absorbs the molecules as it makes contact with them.
- When you apply essential oil to your body, the molecules are absorbed rapidly. In some cases, lymph and blood flow increase, helping provide pain relief and/or promote healing. In other cases, they provide a cleansing effect or block bacteria; others help speed up detoxification.

- When you inhale an essential oil, microscopic molecules travel into your nostrils and pass nerve receptors before being drawn into nasal mucus, where they are dissolved and taken up by your olfactory receptor cells. Once activated, these cells signal the olfactory bulb to send a message to the part of your brain associated with memory, emotion, immune function, hormone function, and basic drives. Now you know why scents are so closely linked to emotions and memories.

Aromas can alter heart rate, blood pressure, and breath rate, and some have the ability to stimulate the release of *enkephalin*, a compound your body uses to stop pain and improve mood. Some aromas prompt the release of the chemical norepinephrine, which then stimulates the immune system and reduces feelings of fatigue. Still others stimulate the *raphe nucleus*, which is found in the brain stem, to release serotonin, producing a sedative action that helps lower blood pressure while relieving issues like insomnia and anxiety. Clearly, when you use aromatherapy, your body's chemistry changes for the better, and that can greatly improve your health overall.

Clary sage essential oil can *even* take on tough bacteria. A study conducted in 2015 proved its ability to kill three strains of *Staphylococcus*, according to researchers at the Medical University of Lodz in Poland.

HOW ESSENTIAL OILS ARE EXTRACTED

Can you make essential oils at home? Since each drop of essential oil contains the full power of pounds of plant matter, the short answer is no. Essential oils are products you'll need to buy, and understanding how they're made can help you identify and choose only the very best.

Why Extraction Method Matters

When shopping for essential oils, you might notice that some companies offer different versions of essential oils made from the same plant species, produced using different extraction methods. The slight differences between these methods can affect the properties of an oil, including volatility, and in some cases, aroma and strength. For instance:

- Certain distilled citrus oils are less stable than expressed oils from the same species, so they deteriorate faster. This isn't necessarily a bad thing; in fact, some of these, such as lemon, may be better for topical application because the distillation process reduces phototoxicity (see Photosensitizing Essential Oils on page 42).
- Distilled patchouli is prized for its aroma, which is warmer and richer than non-distilled types.
- Some CO_2 extracts, including frankincense and myrrh, contain more beneficial molecules than their distilled counterparts, but at higher prices.

Most companies provide information that tells consumers how their essential oils are extracted, and some offer different oils made from the same plants, in which case they typically provide information about the practical benefits of each type. The takeaway? If you're presented with an option, read accompanying literature and/or descriptions carefully to determine which one will best suit your needs.

Common Extraction Methods

Extraction is the term used to describe the process for separating essential oils from other plant matter. Manufacturers use several methods to produce the essential oils that we enjoy so much. Here are three of the most common methods.

Distillation employs water and/or steam to separate essential oils from plant matter. The process takes place inside a large still with a connecting pipe that leads to a condenser from which finished essential oil is siphoned. Many essential oils are made from heavy plant matter that benefits from a long, slow heating process. Examples include cedarwood, chamomile, clary sage, eucalyptus, and lavender.

Expression, also known as cold pressing, is a production method exclusive to citrus essential oils. Because the oils are concentrated inside the fruit's skin, with heavy, protective cell walls around them, this method proves easiest and most economical. Rinds are heated to no more than 50°C (120°F), after which they are pressed. This cool processing ensures that citrus oils retain their fresh, uplifting fragrances.

CO_2 extraction uses carbon dioxide and/or supercritical carbon dioxide to separate essential oils from other plant matter. Since there is no heating involved, oils remain pure and unaltered, meaning the product inside the bottle is as close to the original plant oil as possible. As with distillation and expression, this method produces pure essential oil that is safe to use. In general, all oils extracted via CO_2 are a pleasure to use. Florals such as rose, and spices such as ginger are particularly nice.

SHOPPING FOR ESSENTIAL OILS

When you begin shopping for essential oils, you'll immediately notice differences in price, along with claims that certain brands are "best." Here, you'll gain insight into essential oil labeling, learn about questionable marketing claims, and acquire other important information that will help you become an educated buyer. You can also consult the Essential Oil Brands guide (page 305) at the back of the book for the rundown on 10 of the most popular companies.

Labels

Just like the labels on other products you buy, labels on essential oils contain different types of information. There are no formal regulations governing essential oil labeling, so looking for a few key pieces of information can help you determine whether you're buying good-quality oils. Labels do vary, so don't be alarmed if an item is missing. Just do a little more research, such as by checking out the company's website or contacting them directly, to find the omitted information.

- Ensure that both the common and Latin names of the source plant are included somewhere on the label—for example, a lavender essential oil label should also include the words *Lavandula angustifolia*.
- Unless you are buying a blend or a dilution, such as 10% rose in jojoba oil, the only ingredient listed on the bottle should be the essential oil itself.
- Quality essential oils often include the country of origin, brief usage instructions and/or cautions, and storage info.

Marketing Claims

Some essential oil companies add terminology to their labels as a way of distinguishing their products from others. Claims that certain essential oils are "aromatherapy grade" or "therapeutic grade" are simply marketing claims. This doesn't mean that the manufacturer is out to deceive you; however, you should be aware that there is no governmental regulating body that tests, grades, or certifies essential oils.

When considering a purchase, look for other indicators of quality such as complete labeling information. Accompanying materials often discuss growing methods, harvesting, and other factors that provide insight. Skipping over the marketing claims and simply looking at the rest of the information, quality of packaging, and company reputation may help you avoid confusion.

ESSENTIAL OILS: A MINI GLOSSARY

The terms defined in this mini glossary are among the most commonly used to talk about aromatherapy. You'll find a glossary of medicinal properties at the back of the book.

ABSOLUTE
A highly concentrated oil that has been produced via solvent extraction. Most absolutes are florals, such as rose and jasmine.

ADULTERATED
Essential oil that has been watered down with chemicals or other oils but may still be marketed as pure essential oil.

AROMATHERAPY
The use of aromatic plant materials, primarily essential oils, to alter mood or cognition or to affect psychological or physical well-being. Aromatherapy is often offered as a complementary therapy; however, it is sometimes used as a form of alternative medicine.

CARRIER OIL
A neutral base oil used to dilute essential oils.

DILUTED
When a pure essential oil is blended with a carrier, a lotion, or a liquid such as water, it is said to be diluted.

DISTILLATION
A form of essential oil extraction in which the essential oils are converted to vapor and then condensed back into liquid before bottling.

ESSENTIAL OIL
A concentrated liquid that contains volatile aromatic compounds that have been extracted from plant matter.

EXTRACTION

A means of separating essential oil from other plant matter.

NEAT

Applying an essential oil without first diluting it. You can use your finger or a cotton swab or ball, depending on the size of the area being treated, the amount of oil being used, and what you have on hand.

ORIFICE REDUCER

A clear insert in an essential oil bottle's opening that allows you to dispense oils one drop at a time.

PATCH TEST

A means of testing for sensitivity to an essential oil by placing a drop of diluted essential oil on the inner bend of your elbow. If no irritation occurs after 24 hours, you'll know that the essential oil is safe for use on your skin. Each person who uses an essential oil should first conduct a patch test for sensitivity.

PHOTOSENSITIZING

An essential oil that magnifies the sun's effect and increases your chances of suffering sunburn on the application site.

VOLATILITY

The speed and ease with which an essential oil disperses or evaporates when it comes into contact with the air. Volatility can be affected by temperature, air movement, and other variable factors.

What to Question

While essential oils offer real benefits, it's best to conduct a little research before buying a product. Several companies sell their essential oils via distributorships and multilevel-marketing arrangements. Some of these companies offer excellent products, but it's always smart to ask questions about any statements being made. It's also advisable to avoid products that come with claims that seem too good to be true. Online reviews can help you get a feel for whether a company has a solid reputation in the marketplace.

Additionally, question prices that seem dramatically lower than the prices at competing companies, and look out for anyone selling a variety of essential oils all at the same price. Some types, including jasmine and rose, are quite costly, and pricing ought to reflect that. Rich oils like patchouli, frankincense, and myrrh should cost quite a bit more than those that come from common plants like peppermint, lemon, and mandarin.

What to Avoid

When shopping locally, avoid purchasing essential oils that have been opened, and don't purchase any that look like they've been sitting on a shelf for a long time; dust or sticky residue can be an indicator. Likewise, avoid essential oils that have been stored in a warm location. Many vendors do take proper precautions, but some may not realize that heat can destroy essential oils or may not want to bother taking extra care.

100% PURE THERAPEUTIC GRADE: UNMASKING THE LABEL

There is no question that the quality and purity of essential oil is important. Perhaps that is why some companies continue to use labels claiming that their essential oils are "100% Pure Therapeutic Grade." The liquid inside the bottles may indeed be 100 percent pure essential oil suitable for aromatherapy use, but there is no government or industry organization that grades essential oils as therapeutic.

Instead of relying on marketing claims, check to see whether the essential oils you are considering have been subjected to quantifiable testing via gas chromatography and/or mass spectroscopy. These tests measure the plant constituents contained in essential oils, and they show whether any adulterants are present. Labels that carry the abbreviation GC-MS or GLC-MS indicate that the product in the bottle is pure. This doesn't mean that an oil isn't pure if these abbreviations don't appear on the label; check the company's website to find out.

Another way to look beyond marketing claims is to choose organic essential oils that have also undergone quantifiable testing. Organic producers in the United States are regulated by the U.S. Department of Agriculture (USDA), and products that carry the USDA Organic insignia are certified to be free from herbicides, pesticides, and synthetic substances.

It's best to avoid essential oils that are sold in clear containers rather than dark glass or lined aluminum ones, or have droppers with rubber bulbs. Additionally, avoid essential oils sold in plastic containers, as the oil can dissolve the plastic and become contaminated.

Stay away from anything labeled "perfume oil," "fragrance oil," or "nature identical oil." All of these terms indicate that the substance inside the bottle has probably been adulterated with natural or synthetic constituents.

SHOPPING FOR CARRIER OILS

Carrier oils are usually derived from the seeds, nuts, or kernels of plants. All are 100 percent fat, and though some have a faint, pleasant aroma, it is often barely noticeable. Sometimes referred to as base oils or vegetable oils, carrier oils are used to dilute certain essential oils before application to the skin. Their function is to provide a protective barrier and also to help prevent essential oils from evaporating too quickly upon application.

There are endless essential oil/carrier oil combinations to enjoy, and as the matter of which carrier oil to use with which essential oil is subjective, you'll find that different manufacturers have different recommendations for pairing and creating blends. If I have a personal carrier oil preference for a particular remedy, you'll find it specified in the ingredient list.

Almond oil has a light, nutty, slightly sweet aroma and absorbs rapidly. Moderately priced, it's a good all-around carrier oil to keep on hand. It blends well with almost any essential oil but is particularly nice with warm, spicy essential oils such as clove, frankincense, and myrrh.

Avocado oil has a somewhat sweet smell and a deep, olive-green color. Its texture is full bodied, and it leaves skin feeling well moisturized. Avocado oil is an excellent carrier to use for dry skin, although it is so heavy that you may want to blend it with a lighter oil, like sweet almond, to speed absorption. It is best blended with strong-scented essential oils like lavender and tea tree.

Jojoba oil has a pleasant, light aroma that's less noticeable than that of most nut oils. Light and silky, its texture makes for a very pleasant feel and rapid absorption. While jojoba oil costs a bit more than some other carrier oils, it has a long shelf life and lends itself to a variety of uses. It blends well with any essential oil and is ideal for making massage oils, skin care products, and treatments for hair and scalp conditions.

Safflower oil has a light texture and a faint floral aroma. It is highly nourishing and works well in blends for treating acne, scars, and stretch marks. It is ideal for blending with delicately scented oils such as cedarwood.

Shea butter is rich and nourishing, and lends itself well to use in lotions, conditioners, and thick massage creams. Its fragrance is very light, making it ideal for blending with any essential oil.

USING ESSENTIAL OILS

Essential oils are used in three primary ways: aromatically, topically, and internally. Aromatic and topical are the safest ways to use oils.

Although some people advocate for internal use, claiming that it's the most efficient route of delivery, there are risks involved. For this reason, the remedies in this book are all either aromatic or topical.

If you've been considering ingestion to resolve an issue more quickly, understand that essential oils encounter a variety of bacteria, toxins, and other substances in the digestive system, making it more difficult for them to reach the desired target.

Aromatic Application

Aromatic application occurs whenever essential oils are inhaled, and it is ideal for addressing a wide variety of issues ranging from stress and anxiety to coughing and congestion.

Direct inhalation is ideal for traveling, as no special equipment is needed. You can simply apply a drop or two of a suitable essential oil or blend to a cotton ball, tissue, or handkerchief and inhale deeply. To eliminate the fuss of carrying liquid with you, you can make simple smelling salts (see part 2 for recipes) to take along and inhale as needed.

Indirect inhalation is ideal for treatments at home. Any aromatic application other than direct inhalation is indirect. Here are two popular methods of indirect inhalation:

- *Diffusion* is typically accomplished with a small, purpose-built device called a diffuser that uses a tiny fan or gentle warming to release essential oil molecules into the air. Some diffusers combine the oils with water, creating a gentle mist; others use ultrasonic or nebulizing technology to deliver microscopic particles for easier absorption.
- *Steam inhalation*, or vapor therapy, is accomplished by placing a few drops of essential oil in a bowl of very hot water, and then inhaling the resulting vapors. It is ideal for treating respiratory tract and sinus-related ailments and can be intensified by covering your head and the bowl with a towel, forming a tent that concentrates the vapors. You can also use a humidifier or vaporizer for steam inhalation, or you can add essential oils to a hot bath or shower and breathe deeply. Humidifiers, vaporizers, and baths or showers are less intense than towel tents, making them ideal for treating children under 12 years.

Topical Application

Topical application is exactly what it sounds like: applying essential oils to the skin. There are several ways to accomplish this. Compresses, massage, hand and foot baths, and skin care products are some of the most popular methods for delivering essential oils to the body. So are homemade perfumes blended with a bit of water, carrier oil, and/or alcohol.

Most essential oils need to be diluted in water, oil, or alcohol before being applied to the skin. Only a few are safe

SEVEN MUST-HAVE ESSENTIAL OILS FOR HOME OR ON THE GO

With so many essential oils available, a few things make these seven stand out. Versatility is first and foremost: whether used on their own or combined with others, each offers a multitude of uses. Affordability is second: most of these must-haves are surprisingly inexpensive. Availability is a consideration, too: you'll find these oils online and at health food stores. Finally, each offers mental or emotional benefits as well as physical comfort and healing.

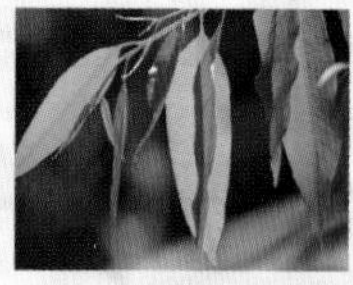

EUCALYPTUS helps clear blocked sinuses quickly, proving effective against colds and allergies alike. It also offers relief for tired feet and overworked muscles.

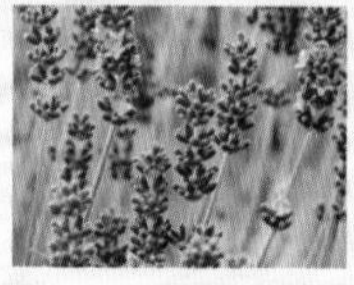

LAVENDER is often described as the Swiss Army knife of the essential oil world, thanks to its ability to fight infection and treat minor injuries. It can be applied neat, so there's no need to bring a carrier oil along. Its relaxing aroma can send you straight to dreamland, no matter how unfamiliar your surroundings.

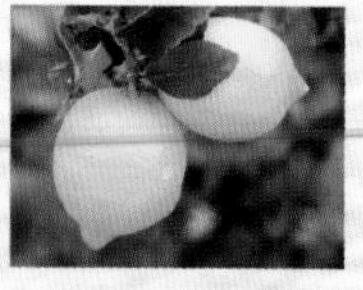

LEMON is an excellent antibacterial that's helpful for treating minor wounds and infections. It also lends itself to a number of household uses, ranging from furniture polish to all-purpose cleaner.

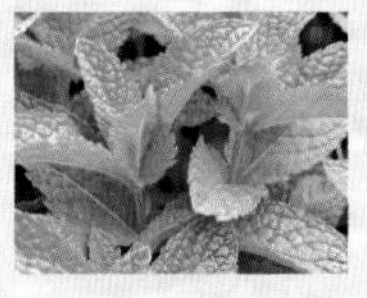

PEPPERMINT has a refreshing aroma that brings mental clarity. It's my go-to for headache relief, and when applied topically, it helps soothe sore muscles in a flash. Peppermint relieves indigestion, too.

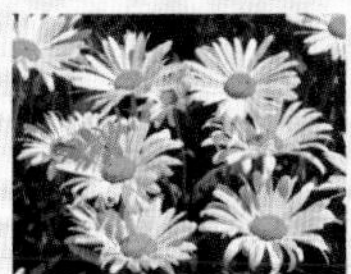

ROMAN CHAMOMILE soothes crying or colicky babies, particularly when blended with lavender. Dry skin, diaper rash, and bee stings are no match for this versatile oil, which also happens to be fantastic for stress relief. Diffuse it to help argumentative kids calm down.

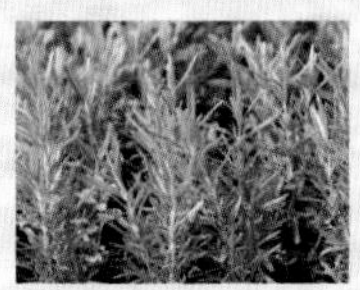

ROSEMARY relaxes muscles while promoting an alert, receptive state of mind. It's my favorite for promoting focus during intense work sessions.

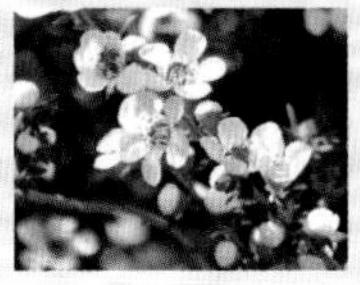

TEA TREE banishes funky odors, eliminates mold and mildew, and treats fungal infections such as athlete's foot. Its ability to stop bug bites from itching makes it a summertime staple.

for neat application, meaning they can be applied directly to the skin without first being diluted. Of course, the remedies in part 2 take this into account.

If you have sensitive skin, it is a good idea to double the amount of carrier oil called for in a remedy just for extra protection. Don't worry—the treatment will be just as effective, and the extra carrier oil will compensate for the reduced amount of essential oil by helping slow down evaporation and increase absorption.

TOOLS AND EQUIPMENT

Essential oil remedies are quick and simple to make, so long as you have a few basic tools on hand. Some of the required equipment is probably in your kitchen, while other items are readily available online and at health food stores. Given frequent use, anything you purchase is more than worth the investment and will pay for itself quickly.

Diffuser You can get a decent diffuser for about $20, although it is possible to drop more than $75 for a top-of-the-line ultrasonic or nebulizing model. If you choose an ultra-affordable glass or soapstone diffuser that calls for candles, choose tea lights with lead-free cotton wicking and paraffin-free wax.

Glass bottles Choose dark-colored glass bottles that protect the light-sensitive compounds in the essential oils from degradation caused by exposure to UV rays. Some of the most useful bottles feature drop-by-drop applicators called *orifice reducers*, which help prevent waste by affording precise control during dispensing. When preparing your remedies, you'll want a few different sizes and types of bottles:

- For small amounts, 15 mL and 30 mL sizes are versatile and practical, allowing you to create and store aromatherapy blends. Larger glass bottles are ideal for storing massage oil, bath oil, and other high-yield remedies: 2-, 4-, 8-, and 16-ounce sizes are common.
- Storage bottles with spray tops or flip tops for easy dispensing in 4-, 8-, and 16-ounce sizes are handy.
- Bottles with twist caps ensure security, and optional glass droppers provide precision. If using droppers, store them separately from bottles containing essential oils, as the vapors from the oils cause flexible dropper tops to degrade.

Glass, ceramic, or stainless steel mixing bowls Because essential oils degrade petroleum products and can therefore "eat" through certain types of plastic, use only glass, ceramic, or stainless steel mixing bowls to formulate remedies. It's nice to have a variety of sizes on hand, but a 2-quart bowl is large enough to handle the recipes in this book that yield larger amounts, such as body lotion and conditioner.

Humidifier/vaporizer A humidifier or vaporizer can be a nice addition to your arsenal, allowing you to deal with issues such as allergies, coughs, and colds while sweetening indoor air.

Liquid measuring cup A 1- to 2-cup glass liquid measuring cup like the one you may already have on hand is essential for precise recipe formulation.

Travel case Protect essential oils while keeping them out of curious little hands by storing them securely inside a purpose-built case. These handy organizers come in different sizes and feature separate compartments for each bottle. You may want to pick one that will accommodate more essential oils than you plan to purchase initially; it's common for a collection to expand as time passes and knowledge increases.

Storing Essential Oils

When you consider the cost per ounce, you'll quickly realize that while essential oils can ultimately make life more affordable, they're far from cheap. Proper storage protects your investment. Here are five tips to follow for safe storage:

1. **Avoid heat and light**. Essential oils are flammable. Do not store them above a woodstove or range. Additionally, avoid direct contact with sunlight, which can adversely affect the essential oil's color and constituents.
2. **Keep away from moisture and oxygen**. Consistent contact with oxygen causes essential oils to deteriorate, rendering them unsuitable for therapeutic purposes. Moisture leads to contamination, so prevent condensation by keeping lids on when the oils are not in use.
3. **Keep bottles full**. The less air space inside a bottle of essential oil, the better. When bottles are about half full,

transfer the remaining amount to a smaller storage bottle to reduce the risk of oxidization.

4. **Keep oils away from children and pets**. While many essential oils are safe for use on children, they can be harmful if swallowed, or cause serious skin problems if applied or inhaled in excessive amounts.
5. **Cap bottles tightly**. Essential oils will evaporate if not tightly capped. Keep your oils tightly capped, not corked. Despite their solid appearance, corks are porous and will allow for slow evaporation over time.

On the Road (or in the Air)

What equipment might you need when traveling? In short, none. Think about where you're going, and make the essential oil blends you'll want to have on hand in advance so they'll be just as convenient as OTC remedies.

Flying to Disney World? You'll contend with crowds at the airport, close quarters on the plane, and jet lag, so bring along essential oil blends that bolster the immune system and help with sleep, such as lavender and eucalyptus.

Heading to the beach or going camping? Think about problems you may have to face such as sunburn, bug bites, or the minor scrapes and bruises that often come from scaling rocks and climbing trees. Poison ivy or poison oak may be an issue during outdoor activities, too.

When planning to bring essential oil remedies to the airport, ensure that any liquids you pack in your carry-on are stored in bottles small enough to meet official safety standards. Larger quantities can be packed in checked luggage, or you can blend your essential oils in a small bottle and then purchase a carrier, such as aloe vera gel for making a sunburn remedy, when you get to your destination.

Knowing what ailments might present themselves when you're traveling can help you determine which essential oils and/or premade remedies to pack. Put everything in one easy-to-access place, and you'll be ready to face challenges without the added stress of digging through your bags.

SAFETY CONSIDERATIONS AND RECOMMENDATIONS

Although essential oils are natural, they are highly concentrated and very potent! Just one drop is enough to stop the burn from a bee sting, soothe muscle pain, or help a cut heal faster. Likewise, one drop can be enough to cause minor skin irritation and severe irritation to eyes and other mucous membranes, so be sure to wash and dry your hands after handling essential oils.

There are no regulated safety standards to follow when using essential oils; however, each oil comes with its own set of precautions. Additionally, there are certain properties to be aware of. Emmenagogues, for example, are often marvelous for easing menstrual discomfort, but because they promote or enhance uterine bleeding, pregnant women should avoid them. Dermal irritants almost always produce immediate skin irritation, and photosensitizing oils can cause mild to severe sunburn.

You'll find notes on common essential oils described in this book that should not be used with the groups outlined below, and you can visit the National Association for Holistic Aromatherapy at NAHA.org/explore-aromatherapy/safety/ to view a more comprehensive list of precautions.

Each remedy in this book includes symbols to let you know if these groups can use it safely, plus specific safety recommendations for people who are suffering from certain illnesses. If you're ever in doubt about safety, it's best to err on the side of caution instead of taking a chance.

Babies and children Use caution when selecting essential oils for babies and children. Many that are fine for diffusion or vapor therapy are too strong for sensitive young skin. Don't apply peppermint, tea tree, or eucalyptus essential oil to anyone under age 6, unless it has been heavily diluted. Be sure to check specific guidelines when considering whether to apply an essential oil to your child's skin.

Pregnant and/or breastfeeding women Pregnant and breastfeeding women should avoid most essential oils. If you are pregnant and considering the use of essential oils, do your research and check labels very carefully.

Seniors Seniors with thin or compromised skin are susceptible to irritation. Clove, lemongrass, thyme, peppermint, tea tree, and eucalyptus are some that may cause problems. Use caution and conduct a patch test before applying essential oils to seniors and others with fragile skin.

PHOTOSENSITIZING ESSENTIAL OILS

Some essential oils are described as photosensitizing or phototoxic, meaning they can lead to a rash or increase the chances of sunburn when the skin on which the oil was applied is exposed to sunlight. You can avoid this effect by applying phototoxic essential oils to your feet or areas normally covered by clothing.

If you do use a phototoxic essential oil on an exposed area of skin, you will need to avoid sun exposure for the periods of time given below. If you have very fair skin or usually sunburn when you go out without sunscreen, stay on the safe side by doubling the times listed.

12 HOURS

Tangerine and blends containing it

24 HOURS

Ginger, grapefruit, lemon, mandarin, orange, and blends containing them

48 HOURS

Bergamot and blends containing it, unless labeled "Bergaptene-Free" or "Bergamot FCF"

72 HOURS

Lime and blends containing it

Don't make the mistake of adding one of these oils to lotion and applying it before going into the sun in hopes of tanning faster. You'll burn instead, causing pain and damaging your skin.

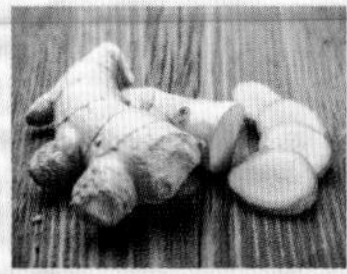

Ginger

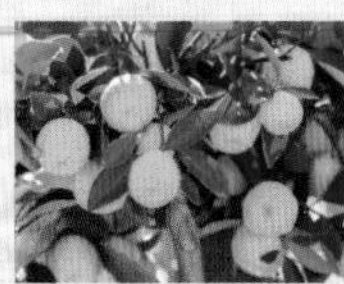

Mandarin

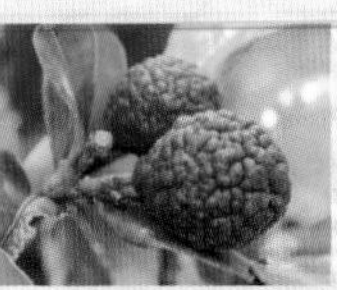

Bergamot

Pets The use of essential oils on pets is controversial and something I've chosen not to focus on in this book. Although some essential oils can be toxic to pets, and cats in particular, pet owners can use oils safely by taking precautions to make sure their pets don't touch, ingest, or inhale the vapors of these oils directly. I use essential oils with my cats, dogs, chickens, and horses, but it's a personal decision that must be entered into knowledgeably. If you're interested, talk to your veterinarian about which oils are safest to use around or directly with pets.

WHAT'S NEXT?

In part 2 you'll find a wealth of remedies for a variety of health issues that you and your family may encounter whether at home, on vacation, or anywhere else you may find yourself. A list of A-to-Z ailments with step-by-step treatments makes it easy to find what you're looking for and get back on the road to health—fast. And because knowledge is power, part 3 offers concise profiles of 50 of the most common, versatile, and largely affordable essential oils and their properties. Why 50? Because while many of the most popular essential oil storage and carrying cases feature compartments for 30 essential oil bottles, not everyone wants to use the same ones. Knowing about 50 essential oils expands your knowledge base and gives you plenty of options to choose from. Of course, you also have the option of choosing all 50 of these or adding more of the hundreds of oils available.

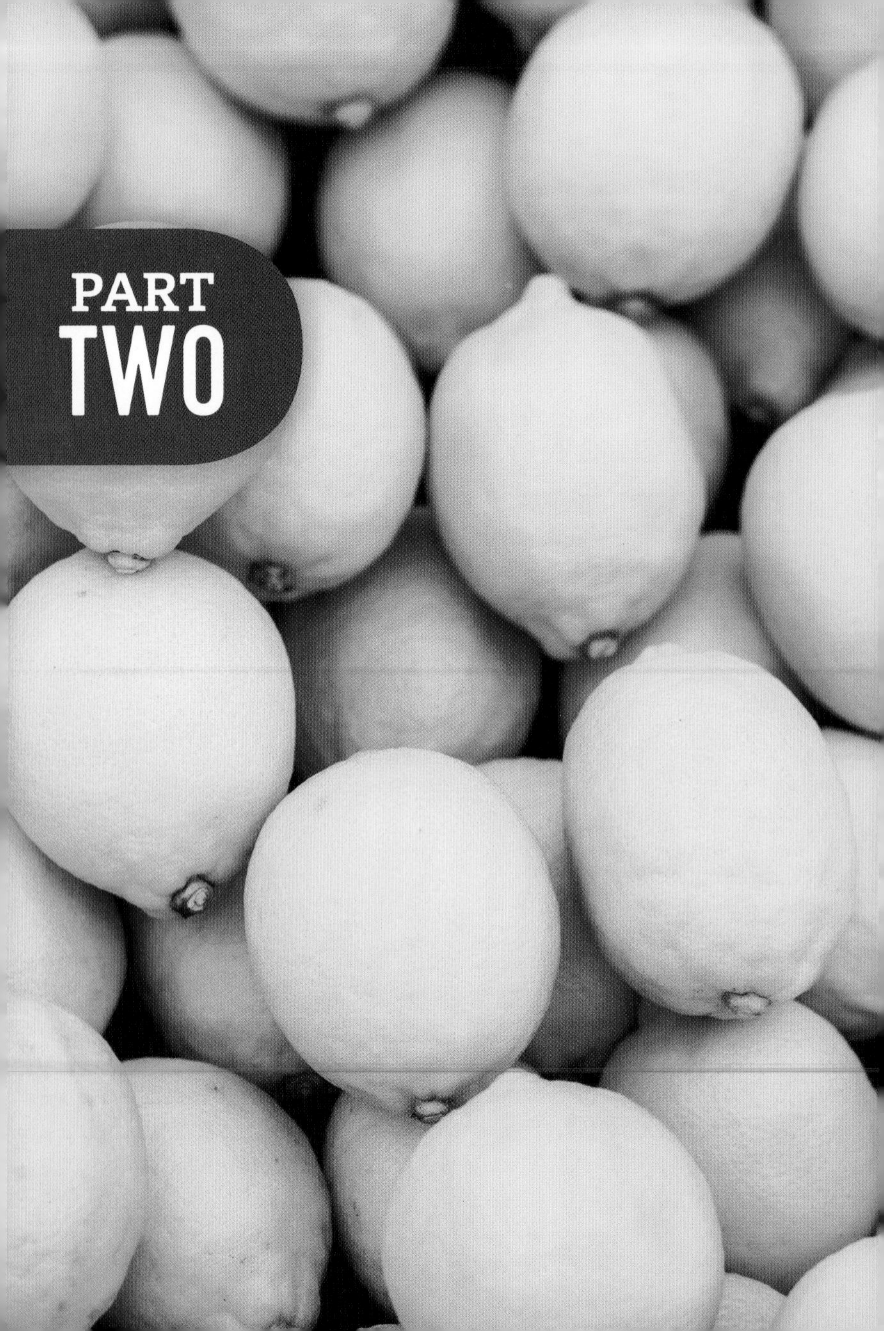

PART TWO

Ailments & Remedies

Essential oils can be used as alternatives to over-the-counter (OTC) drugs, letting you treat a wide range of ailments quickly, easily, and completely naturally. You'll find relief for skin problems ranging from acne to psoriasis here plus powerful remedies for issues like athlete's foot and ringworm. Cold and flu symptoms are no match for essential oils, which often bring relief via vapor therapy or simple diffusion.

Whether you're looking for a way to get rid of hiccups or stop the burning itch that accompanies an unfortunate run-in with poison ivy, finding it is as simple as making your way through this A-to-Z list of ailments and then choosing one of the corresponding remedies.

Every remedy includes a few concise notes for safe, effective use. You'll see upfront whether the treatment is inhaled or applied topically, plus you can see at a glance whether it is safe for children. If you don't see a note about age—that is, 2+ years, 6+ years, or 12+ years—then you know that the oils used in the remedy are considered safe for children of all ages. If a treatment can cause photosensitivity and increase your risk of sunburn, you'll know before taking the time to read further.

SAFETY KEY

Aromatic	Topical	May Cause Photosensitivity	Safe for Children Ages		
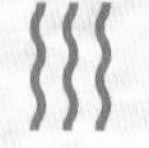	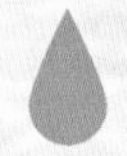	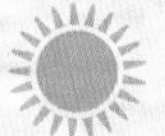	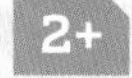	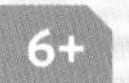	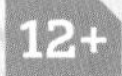

A list of ingredients is next, followed by step-by-step instructions. Each remedy includes a quick note about how it should be stored for convenience or lasting potency, if applicable. Additionally, every remedy offers a final tip that might include information about modifying a particular remedy so that it's safe for those who shouldn't use it as written, such as young children or pregnant women. Other tips cover alternate methods for using the essential oils or recipes. And, in case you don't have certain oils on hand, some of the tips suggest substitutions.

Essential oils are best for treating minor conditions, and they can often complement remedies prescribed by your doctor. As you'll soon discover, just a little bit of essential oil goes a long way. If your symptoms are serious, or if you have a major injury such as a deep cut that needs stitches, seek medical help right away. Finally, remember that some essential oils interact with drugs. If you are taking a prescription of any kind, even for an unrelated problem, check with your physician before using even the simplest remedy.

ABSCESS

Occurring during the last stage of tissue infections, abscesses can occur anywhere on the body. Red and swollen, they are hot to the touch and painful for the sufferer. Since skin resists the spread of infection, it acts as a barrier, trapping pus inside. In case of a superficial abscess located on the limbs or trunk, tea tree, lavender, and chamomile essential oils can help by working to stop the infection while providing pain relief. Seek medical attention if the abscess is larger than half an inch across.

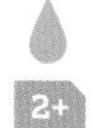

Chamomile, Lavender, and Tea Tree Compress

MAKES ABOUT 8 OUNCES

60 drops lavender essential oil

40 drops chamomile essential oil

20 drops tea tree essential oil

1 cup steaming hot (not boiling) water

1. In a small bottle with a tight-fitting lid and an orifice reducer, combine the lavender, chamomile, and tea tree essential oils. Secure the lid and shake well to blend.
2. Pour the water into a wide bowl and add 12 drops of the oil blend to the water. ➛

Chamomile, Lavender, and Tea Tree Compress continued

3. Swish a cotton washcloth through the water and wring it out completely. Apply the cloth to the abscess and leave it in place until the cloth cools. Then wet the cloth again and reapply. Continue to reapply for at least 15 minutes.
4. Repeat three times daily for three days. Discontinue the hot compresses if the abscess drains before the treatment cycle ends.

STORAGE Keep in a cool, dark place.

TIP For those 12 years and up, add 20 drops of thyme essential oil to the blend if you have it on hand, and increase the amount of blended oil used per treatment to 14 drops. This can help speed the draining process. After draining occurs, keep the area dry and clean. See your doctor if you notice any signs of infection while treating.

Tea Tree Neat Treatment

MAKES 1 TREATMENT

1 drop tea tree essential oil

Apply the tea tree essential oil directly to the abscess. Repeat two to three times daily for three days. Discontinue the application if the abscess drains before the treatment cycle ends.

TIP For children under 12 years, dilute the tea tree by combining it with an equal amount of carrier oil. My go-to carriers include jojoba and sweet almond.

ACNE

The pain and discomfort of acne are bad enough; the embarrassment of visible blemishes makes it even worse. Essential oils with antiseptic and antibacterial properties are effective, budget-friendly alternatives to expensive creams, lotions, or pills. Most acne sufferers find that these remedies reduce inflammation and redness, which helps improve the appearance of affected areas. Essential oils with strong antiseptic and antibacterial properties are best for acne: lavender, clove, tea tree, oregano, and rosemary.

Clove Balm

MAKES ABOUT ¼ OUNCE

1½ teaspoons sweet almond oil

12 drops clove essential oil

1. In a small bottle with a tight-fitting lid and an orifice reducer, combine the sweet almond and clove essential oils. Secure the lid and shake well to blend.
2. Wash and dry your face. Then, using a cotton swab, apply one or two drops of the balm to the affected area. Repeat once or twice daily as needed.

STORAGE Keep in a cool, dark place.

TIP This remedy is especially effective for use on painful pimples, but it can also help put a stop to emerging breakouts. Use as a spot treatment only.

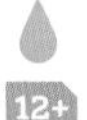

Natural Acne Gel

MAKES ABOUT 2 OUNCES

¼ cup aloe vera gel

12 drops geranium essential oil

10 drops lavender essential oil

8 drops tea tree essential oil

1. In a small jar with a tight-fitting lid, combine the aloe gel with the geranium, lavender, and tea tree essential oils. Stir well with a thin utensil.
2. Wash and dry your face. Using a cotton ball, apply the gel, focusing on blemishes and avoiding the eye area. Repeat twice daily.

STORAGE Keep in a cool, dark place or in the refrigerator for a cooling sensation with each use.

TIP Once acne clears, prevent recurrences by applying a thin layer of the gel to clean, dry, acne-prone areas once daily.

Lavender Zit Zapper

MAKES 1 TREATMENT

1 drop lavender essential oil

Using a cotton swab, gently dab the lavender essential oil onto the pimple. Repeat once or twice daily as needed.

TIP If you're all out of lavender or want to use something a little stronger, try tea tree. The downside of tea tree is that it can cause sensitive facial skin to dry out fast, so keep an eye on it.

ALLERGIES

Congestion, runny nose, nasal itching, and sneezing are some of the most irritating and persistent allergy symptoms. While there is no cure for allergies, essential oils can help alleviate the symptoms and make the sufferer more comfortable. Make your treatment plan more effective by getting to the root of the problem and addressing indoor allergy culprits such as dust, pet dander, and chemicals found in personal care products, scented candles, household cleaners, and the like. If you suspect that mold is part of the problem, consider hiring a specialist to check your home.

Chamomile-Eucalyptus Diffusion

MAKES 1 TREATMENT

3 drops Roman chamomile essential oil

3 drops eucalyptus essential oil

Following the manufacturer's instructions, add the Roman chamomile and eucalyptus essential oils to your diffuser. Run the diffuser nearby. Repeat every two to three hours or as needed.

TIP This blend is good for vapor therapy, too. Use it in a humidifier or vaporizer, or add the Roman chamomile and eucalyptus essential oils to your bath.

Tea Tree Room Spray

MAKES ABOUT 23 OUNCES

2¾ cups distilled or purified water

1 tablespoon tea tree essential oil

1. In a large bottle with a fine-mist spray top, combine the water and tea tree essential oil and secure the top. Shake well before each use.
2. Spritz potential allergy sources including furniture, vents, carpets, appliances, and bedding.

STORAGE Keep in a convenient location if using frequently; otherwise, keep in a cool, dark place.

TIP Use a few spritzes of this solution each day to keep allergens under control. You can also use this spray as a natural alternative to commercial mold preventives by spritzing down the bath/shower area after each use.

Peppermint Salve

MAKES ABOUT ⅓ OUNCE

2 teaspoons carrier oil

4 drops peppermint essential oil

1. In a small bottle with a tight-fitting lid and an orifice reducer, combine the carrier oil with the peppermint essential oil. Secure the lid and shake well to blend.
2. Apply three to five drops of the blend to the base of your neck. Repeat twice daily whenever allergy symptoms are present.

STORAGE Keep in a cool, dark place.

TIP When children younger than 6 years suffer from indoor allergy symptoms, use lavender or spearmint essential oil instead of peppermint. Although they're milder remedies, they can help clear stuffy sinuses.

ANXIETY

Persistent nervousness or fear, compulsive or repetitive behaviors, and a strong desire to avoid social situations are some of the most troublesome signs and symptoms of anxiety. While severe cases call for professional help, essential oils can help ease mild anxiety. Some essential oils, such as lavender and chamomile, lead to feelings of physical and mental relaxation. Others, including rosemary and eucalyptus, reduce anxiety while promoting a sense of alertness and overall well-being. Try different remedies to suit the time of day and support the energy level you desire.

Bergamot Diffusion

MAKES 1 TREATMENT

5 or 6 drops bergamot essential oil

Following the manufacturer's instructions, add the bergamot essential oil to your diffuser. Run the diffuser for 30 minutes one to three times daily.

TIP Help children under 6 years deal with anxiety by diffusing lavender instead of bergamot.

Chamomile-Lavender Massage Oil

MAKES ABOUT 4 OUNCES

½ cup jojoba oil

½ teaspoon vitamin E

16 drops lavender essential oil

16 drops Roman chamomile essential oil

1. In a small bottle or jar with a tight-fitting lid, combine the jojoba oil, vitamin E, and lavender and Roman chamomile essential oils. Secure the lid and shake well to blend.
2. Using just enough massage oil to reduce friction, massage your hands and wrists, temples, feet, or nape of neck. (The amount to use depends on the size of the area you're focusing on.)
3. After application, massage until the oil is completely absorbed. Breathe deeply and try to focus on relaxing.

STORAGE Keep in a cool, dark place.

TIP Besides helping ease anxiety and promote deep relaxation, this massage oil is wonderfully moisturizing. Try it on rough skin or apply a drop to dry, ragged cuticles. You can promote peaceful sleep by using a teaspoon of the massage oil to moisturize your entire body after an evening shower or bath.

Rosemary-Eucalyptus Spray

MAKES ABOUT 8 OUNCES

1 cup distilled or purified water

12 drops rosemary essential oil

6 drops eucalyptus essential oil

1. In a small bottle with a fine-mist spray top, combine the water with the rosemary and eucalyptus essential oils and secure the top. Shake well before each use.
2. Spritz the air nearby three to five times every hour or less frequently, as needed.

STORAGE Keep in a convenient location if using frequently; otherwise, keep in a cool, dark place.

TIP This spray makes a nice, all-purpose air freshener that can take the place of chemical-laden commercial blends. You can make it even more invigorating by adding 12 drops of lemon and/or peppermint essential oil to the blend.

ASTHMA

Asthma leads to an ongoing battle with wheezing and low-level congestion that can make life seem miserable. During asthma attacks brought on by allergic reactions to airborne allergens, stress, and food, the lungs must fight to push air through irritated, swollen bronchial passages. Essential oils with antihistamine and decongestant properties can help ease wheezing; peppermint, ginger, geranium, and marjoram are among the best for clearing lungs between attacks. Essential oils that reduce stress and promote relaxation are also good for asthma. Lavender and frankincense are two to try, since they facilitate emotional balance while helping keep the airways clear. ➛

Lavender Smelling Salts

MAKES ABOUT ½ OUNCE

1 tablespoon Epsom salt or Dead Sea salt

3 drops lavender essential oil

1. In a small jar with a tight-fitting lid, combine the salt with the lavender essential oil. Secure the lid and shake well to blend.
2. To use, inhale deeply from the jar as needed to help keep lungs clear.

STORAGE Keep in a convenient location.

TIP Essential oils evaporate over time, so it's a good idea to refresh your smelling salts periodically. Add another 3 drops of lavender when you notice the scent beginning to fade.

Rosemary-Lemon Vapor Treatment

MAKES 1 TREATMENT

2 cups steaming hot (not boiling) water

3 drops rosemary essential oil

2 drops lemon essential oil

1. Pour the water into a shallow bowl and add the rosemary and lemon essential oils.
2. Sitting comfortably in front of the bowl, drape a towel over your head and the bowl, creating a tent that concentrates the steam and vapors. Breathe deeply until the water cools and the vapors subside, emerging for cool air as needed. Repeat once or twice daily.

TIP As an alternative to the vapor tent for children under 12 years, diffuse the essential oils a few feet away from the activity area or in the child's bedroom. A vaporizer or humidifier is another option.

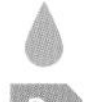

Breathe Easy Aromatherapy Massage Oil

MAKES ABOUT 2 OUNCES

4 tablespoons jojoba oil

6 drops geranium essential oil

3 drops lavender essential oil

3 drops marjoram essential oil

3 drops frankincense essential oil

1. In a small bottle or jar with a tight-fitting lid, combine the jojoba oil with the geranium, lavender, marjoram, and frankincense essential oils. Secure the lid and shake well to blend.
2. Rub generously on the back and chest between asthma attacks. The amount to use depends on the person's size—for example, start with ¼ teaspoon for a 2-year-old and increase the amount incrementally for older children and adults.

STORAGE Keep in a convenient location if using frequently; otherwise, keep in a cool, dark place.

TIP This mild remedy is ideal for children between the ages of 2 and 6. You can double the amount of essential oils in the recipe if using for older children or adults.

ATHLETE'S FOOT

Uncomfortably itchy and highly contagious, athlete's foot usually begins between the toes. At the first sign of discomfort, use a remedy that contains antifungal essential oils to prevent it from worsening. Strong antifungal agents, tea tree, lemon, and lavender are among the best essential oils for athlete's foot. Help your feet heal faster by keeping them clean and dry and by exposing them to air and light as often as you can.

Lavender–Tea Tree Massage Oil

MAKES ABOUT ⅓ OUNCE

2 teaspoons safflower oil

20 drops tea tree essential oil

10 drops lavender essential oil

5 drops lemon essential oil

1. In a small bottle with a tight-fitting lid and an orifice reducer, combine the safflower oil with the tea tree, lavender, and lemon essential oils. Secure the lid and shake well to blend.
2. Apply 5 drops to a cotton ball and swab the affected areas. Use more if needed, and repeat the treatment two to three times daily.

STORAGE Keep in a convenient location if using frequently; otherwise, keep in a cool, dark place.

TIP In a pinch, use either tea tree or lavender neat by using a cotton swab to apply a drop or two to the affected area two to three times daily.

Refreshing Athlete's Foot Spray

MAKES ABOUT 8 OUNCES

8 ounces distilled or purified water

20 drops tea tree essential oil

15 drops lavender essential oil

10 drops peppermint essential oil

10 drops rosemary essential oil

1. In a small bottle with a fine-mist spray top, combine the water with the tea tree, lavender, peppermint, and rosemary essential oils. Secure the top and shake well to blend.
2. Wash and dry your feet and spritz thoroughly, focusing on problem areas. Allow your feet to dry naturally before putting on socks and shoes.

STORAGE Keep in a convenient location if using frequently; otherwise, keep in a cool, dark place.

TIP Spritz inside footwear each evening. Besides targeting bacteria inside, it eliminates odors and helps keep your athlete's foot from getting worse.

Clove Foot Powder

MAKES ABOUT 8 OUNCES

1 cup baking soda

20 drops clove essential oil

1. In a glass or stainless-steel sugar shaker, combine the baking soda with the clove essential oil. Secure the top and shake well from side to side to blend.
2. After bathing or showering, apply a dusting of the powder to your feet. Repeat once or twice daily.

STORAGE Keep in a convenient location if using frequently; otherwise, keep in a cool, dark place.

TIP If you don't have clove essential oil, make this treatment with tea tree or lavender instead.

BACK PAIN

Sitting for hours on end can lead to back pain, and so can overuse. Essential oils work best for minor to moderate discomfort, bringing relief while you get to the root of the problem. When spasms are present, massaging with blends that include lavender, Roman chamomile, or rosemary may help. For simple soreness, try remedies containing peppermint or ginger. If you have injured yourself, be sure to see your doctor to determine the best course of action.

Ginger Neat Treatment

MAKES 1 TREATMENT

4 drops ginger essential oil

Apply the ginger essential oil directly to the painful area. Repeat every four to six hours, as needed.

TIP If you don't have ginger on hand, use peppermint or spearmint instead.

Minty Juniper-Thyme Compress

MAKES 1 TREATMENT

1 teaspoon carrier oil

10 drops peppermint essential oil

10 drops juniper essential oil

5 drops thyme essential oil

1. In the palm of your hand, combine the carrier oil with the peppermint, juniper, and thyme essential oils. Rub your hands together briefly and then apply the blend to the painful area.
2. Cover the site with a soft cloth, then relax with a warm (not hot) heating pad over it for 15 to 30 minutes. Repeat once or twice daily as needed.

TIP This compress works well for muscle pain and minor sprains, too.

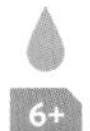

6+

Lavender and Clary Sage Rub

MAKES ABOUT 4 OUNCES

4 ounces safflower oil

25 drops clary sage essential oil

25 drops lavender essential oil

1. In a small bottle with a tight-fitting lid, combine the safflower oil with the clary sage and lavender essential oils. Secure the lid and shake well to blend.
2. Apply enough to cover the painful portion of the back. Massage well and repeat every three to four hours as needed.

STORAGE Keep in a cool, dark place.

TIP Make a similar pain rub for young children by substituting the clary sage with spearmint or Roman chamomile.

BAD BREATH

Bad breath is an unpleasant condition with a number of causes, but it can happen even when you practice good dental hygiene. Commercial remedies and gum often contain undesirable chemicals and artificial sweeteners. Essential oils have the advantage of being all natural—they kill germs while freshening your breath without all the chemicals. Plus, they cost just a few pennies to make.

Orange-Clove Rinse

MAKES ABOUT 8 OUNCES

8 ounces distilled or purified water

3 drops clove essential oil

2 drops orange essential oil

1. In a small bottle with a tight-fitting lid, combine the water with the clove and orange essential oils and secure the lid. Shake well before each use.
2. Rinse your mouth with ½ tablespoon of this solution, taking care not to swallow. Swish for 30 seconds, then spit. Repeat as needed.

STORAGE Keep in a cool, dark place.

TIP Prefer minty breath? Use 6 drops of peppermint or spearmint instead of clove and orange.

Ginger Breath Spray

MAKES ABOUT 2 OUNCES

2 ounces distilled or purified water

1 drop ginger essential oil

1. In a small bottle with a fine-mist spray top, combine the water with the ginger essential oil and secure the top. Shake well before each use.
2. Spray the inside of your mouth with a single spritz of breath spray, taking care not to swallow. Your mouth will absorb the mixture quickly. Repeat as needed. →

Ginger Breath Spray continued

STORAGE Keep in a convenient location.

TIP Add a drop of cinnamon, orange, or lemon essential oil to create a signature breath spray. This spritz also makes a handy air freshener for the car, restroom, and other areas prone to funkiness.

BEE STING

Bee stings are shockingly painful. Left untreated, they can lead to serious swelling and redness. Many essential oils are suitable for treating bee stings; the remedies described here call for lavender and Roman chamomile, so they're safe to use on kids. Be sure to remove the stinger if it's still in place. If you think that you or your child might be having an allergic reaction to a bee sting, skip the essential oil and get to the doctor right away. If that reaction includes difficulty breathing or swallowing, call 911.

Roman Chamomile Compress

MAKES 1 TREATMENT

4 ounces cold water

4 ounces ice

4 drops Roman chamomile essential oil

1. In a shallow bowl, stir to combine the water, ice, and Roman chamomile essential oil.

2. Use a cloth to apply the mixture to the affected area, wringing out the cloth and repeating until all the liquid is gone. Repeat two to three times daily until the pain and swelling subside.

TIP If you can't make a compress, apply 1 drop of carrier oil and 1 drop of Roman chamomile essential oil to the sting site, cover it with a soft cloth and then apply an ice pack, if possible. Try to leave the pack in place for 10 to 15 minutes.

Lavender-Chamomile Poultice

MAKES ABOUT ⅓ OUNCE

2 teaspoons apple cider vinegar

8 drops lavender essential oil

8 drops Roman chamomile essential oil

1. In a small bottle or jar with a tight-fitting lid, combine the apple cider vinegar with the lavender and Roman chamomile essential oils. Secure the lid and shake well to blend.
2. Apply ¼ teaspoon of the blend to a cotton ball.
3. Place the cotton ball on the affected area and hold or tape it in place, leaving it in position for 10 minutes. Repeat four times daily.

STORAGE Keep in a cool, dark place.

TIP In a pinch? Use lemon juice or any type of vinegar if you don't have apple cider vinegar.

Soothing Lemongrass-Clove Spray

MAKES ABOUT 4 OUNCES

4 ounces alcohol-free witch hazel

10 drops lemongrass essential oil

15 drops clove essential oil

1. In a small bottle with a fine-mist spray top, combine the witch hazel with the lemongrass and clove essential oils and secure the top. Shake well before each use.
2. Apply a single spritz to the bee sting, and repeat the treatment two to three times daily.

STORAGE Keep in a cool, dark place.

TIP This spray is good for pain relief, but it also has strong antifungal action. Try it for foot odor and athlete's foot.

BLACKHEADS

Deeply embedded blackheads can be tough to eliminate. Essential oils such as tea tree, lavender, lemongrass, and juniper can help clear them up while addressing redness and inflammation. Like conventional remedies, these natural ones take time to work. Make essential oils part of your skin care routine, and you'll likely see a big difference over the course of a week or two.

Juniper-Lemongrass Salt Scrub

MAKES 1 TREATMENT

1 teaspoon Dead Sea salt

1 teaspoon honey

2 drops juniper essential oil

2 drops lemongrass essential oil

1. In a small bowl, combine the salt and honey with the juniper and lemongrass essential oils. Stir well with a thin utensil.
2. Wet your face and use your fingertips to apply the entire treatment. Use gentle circular motions to massage your face, focusing primarily on affected areas.
3. Rinse well and pat dry. Repeat twice weekly.

TIP If you don't have juniper and lemongrass essential oils, try a blend of 2 drops each of lavender and tea tree.

Clary Sage Cream

MAKES ABOUT 1 OUNCE

1 (1-ounce) container oil-free facial moisturizer

25 drops clary sage essential oil

1. Open the container and remove the seal. Add the clary sage essential oil directly to the container. Stir well with a thin utensil.
2. Apply a small amount of the cream to the affected area twice daily, using just enough for your face to absorb it completely. ➛

Clary Sage Cream continued

STORAGE Store as you would any other moisturizer.

TIP If your favorite oil-free moisturizer comes in a larger or smaller size, adjust the amount of clary sage essential oil accordingly—for example, use 50 drops for a 2-ounce container of moisturizer.

Citrus–Tea Tree Balm

MAKES ABOUT 4 OUNCES

4 ounces aloe vera gel

20 drops tea tree essential oil

10 drops lemon essential oil

10 drops mandarin essential oil

1. In a small jar with a tight-fitting lid, combine the aloe gel with the tea tree, lemon, and mandarin essential oils. Stir well with a thin utensil.
2. Apply ½ teaspoon to your face. Allow the blend to absorb completely before applying any cosmetics. Use once or twice daily.

STORAGE Keep in a cool, dark place.

TIP If you don't have lemon or mandarin essential oil or if you plan to spend time in the sun, you can substitute the citrus oils with an equal amount of lavender. Use 20 drops of lavender if replacing both citrus oils, or 10 drops if replacing just one.

BLISTER

A day of shopping or walking around a theme park can cause chafing that leads to blisters. A day of gardening or using woodworking tools can also cause painful blisters on the hands. While essential oils can sting for a moment when applied to blisters, they can also help promote faster healing and prevent infection. Lavender, tea tree, and myrrh are three of the best to try.

Lavender-Chamomile Footbath

MAKES 1 TREATMENT

1 gallon steaming hot (not boiling) water

½ cup Epsom salt

3 drops lavender essential oil

3 drops Roman chamomile essential oil

1. Fill a basin with the hot water. Dissolve the salt, then add the lavender and Roman chamomile essential oils.
2. Soak your feet until the water cools. Dry off by patting your feet with a soft towel. Repeat once daily while the blisters are healing.

TIP Rejuvenate your entire body while helping blisters heal. Add 2 cups of Epsom salt and 12 drops of each essential oil to a bathtub filled with hot water. A whole-body bath may also be easier for restless children to tolerate than a footbath.

Lavender Neat Treatment

MAKES 1 TREATMENT

1 drop lavender essential oil

1. Wash the affected area in warm, soapy water and pat dry.
2. Use a clean finger or cotton swab to apply the lavender essential oil directly to the blister. Repeat two to three times daily until the blister is gone.

TIP Tea tree or myrrh can also be used as a neat treatment on a blister; simply follow the same protocol.

Eucalyptus-Helichrysum Salve

MAKES ABOUT 1 OUNCE

1 ounce aloe vera gel

15 drops helichrysum essential oil

10 drops eucalyptus essential oil

1. In a small jar with a tight-fitting lid, combine the aloe gel with the helichrysum and eucalyptus essential oils. Stir well with a thin utensil.
2. Apply a pea-size amount to each blister. Repeat two to three times daily or as needed.

STORAGE Keep in a cool, dark place.

TIP If you don't have helichrysum, you can replace it with an equal amount of lavender.

BLOATING OR CRAMPING

The moodiness that accompanies PMS is bad enough; uncomfortable bloating and painful cramping make matters even worse. Instead of going for an OTC pain reliever, give soothing essential oils a try. Lavender, marjoram, and clary sage help stop the muscle contractions associated with cramping while offering pain relief. Lemon, mint, and grapefruit help banish bloating.

Mandarin-Ginger Compress

MAKES 1 TREATMENT

1 teaspoon carrier oil

5 drops mandarin essential oil

5 drops ginger essential oil

1. In the palm of your hand, combine the carrier oil with the mandarin and ginger essential oils. Rub your hands together briefly and apply the blend to your lower abdomen.
2. Massage gently for 1 minute, then cover the area with a soft cloth. Apply a warm heating pad and relax for 15 to 20 minutes. Repeat once or twice daily.

TIP Try this treatment even if you don't have a heating pad. Make it more effective by spending at least 15 minutes in a hot bath before applying the blend and relaxing.

Relaxing Bath Blend

MAKES 1 TREATMENT

1 cup Epsom salt

6 drops lavender essential oil

4 drops marjoram essential oil

3 drops clary sage essential oil

1. Draw a hot bath. Dissolve the salt and add the lavender, marjoram, and clary sage essential oils.
2. Spend 20 to 30 minutes soaking.

TIP This treatment is also useful after a long flight, helping eliminate stress while soothing muscles that have been stuck in one position for hours. Make it to-go by combining the Epsom salt with the essential oils in a resealable baggie.

Peppermint-Citrus Massage Oil

MAKES ABOUT 4 OUNCES

4 ounces jojoba oil

12 drops peppermint essential oil

6 drops grapefruit essential oil

6 drops lemon essential oil

1. In a small bottle or jar with a tight-fitting lid, combine the jojoba oil with the peppermint, grapefruit, and lemon essential oils. Secure the lid and shake well to blend.
2. Apply ½ teaspoon of the oil to the lower abdominal area, using gentle kneading motions. Repeat two to three times daily for relief from bloating.

STORAGE Keep in a cool, dark place.

TIP If you have just one of the citrus oils, use 12 drops instead of 6.

BODY ODOR

Most commercial deodorants contain a whole slew of toxic chemicals, so it makes sense to cut back on their use. What to do instead? Essential oils can tackle even the toughest case of BO. These quick remedies offer fantastic fragrances and are inexpensive to make. Patchouli, lavender, bergamot, rosemary, and tea tree are some of my deodorizing favorites, but you can easily substitute with whichever oils you have on hand. For really tough body odor, choose essential oils with antibacterial or bactericidal properties.

Vetiver–Ylang-Ylang Deodorant Gel

MAKES 2 OUNCES

2 ounces aloe vera gel

20 drops vetiver essential oil

15 drops ylang-ylang essential oil

1. In a small jar with a tight-fitting lid, combine the aloe gel with the vetiver and ylang-ylang essential oils. Stir well with a thin utensil.
2. After showering, apply ¼ teaspoon of the blend to each underarm. Repeat once daily, or more often if needed.

STORAGE Keep in a cool, dark place. →

Vetiver–Ylang-Ylang Deodorant Gel continued

TIP Instead of vetiver and ylang-ylang, you can make this gel with 20 drops lavender and 10 drops tea tree essential oils.

Tea Tree Body Powder

MAKES ABOUT 8 OUNCES

½ cup baking soda

½ cup non-GMO cornstarch

20 drops tea tree essential oil

1. In a glass or stainless-steel sugar shaker, combine the baking soda, cornstarch, and tea tree essential oil. Secure the top and shake well from side to side to blend.
2. Shake about ½ teaspoon of the powder onto a cloth and apply to your underarms and any other problem areas. Use once or twice daily as needed.

STORAGE Keep in a cool, dark place.

TIP This powder works wonders on stinky shoes, too. Just shake a little into each shoe after wearing.

Minty Lavender-Rosemary Deodorant Spray

MAKES ABOUT 8 OUNCES

7½ ounces distilled or purified water

½ ounce rubbing alcohol

20 drops peppermint essential oil

20 drops lavender essential oil

20 drops rosemary essential oil

1. In a small bottle with a fine-mist spray top, combine the water and rubbing alcohol with the peppermint, lavender, and rosemary essential oils and secure the top. Shake well before each use.
2. Spritz your underarms once or twice daily as needed.

STORAGE Keep in a cool, dark place.

TIP This spray makes a wonderfully refreshing all-over body spray. It's a pleasant room freshener, too.

BRONCHITIS

Inflamed bronchial passages result in breathlessness and a hacking cough. Essential oils can complement traditional therapies, but they aren't meant to replace antibiotics and other prescribed medical treatments for this condition. Soothing frankincense, eucalyptus, and marjoram are just a few oils that can bring relief from symptoms.

Frankincense Vapor

MAKES 1 TREATMENT

2 cups steaming hot (not boiling) water

2 drops frankincense essential oil

1. Pour the water into a shallow bowl and add the frankincense essential oil. →

Frankincense Vapor continued

2. Sitting comfortably in front of the bowl, drape a towel over your head and the bowl, creating a tent that concentrates the steam and vapors. Breathe deeply until the water cools and the vapors subside, emerging for cool air as needed. Repeat once or twice daily.

TIP As an alternative to the vapor tent for children under 12 years, diffuse the essential oil a few feet away from the activity area or in the child's bedroom.

Breathe Easy Balm

MAKES ABOUT 1 OUNCE

1 ounce jojoba oil

12 drops eucalyptus essential oil

6 drops peppermint essential oil

5 drops thyme essential oil

1. In a small bottle or jar with a tight-fitting lid, combine the jojoba oil with the eucalyptus, peppermint, and thyme essential oils. Secure the lid and shake well to blend.
2. Apply 5 or 6 drops of the blend to the chest and throat area three or four times daily while symptoms persist.

STORAGE Keep in a cool, dark place.

TIP This balm is fantastic for treating congestion anytime; you may want to mix up a batch to keep on hand during cold season.

BRUISE

Bruises aren't just a cosmetic problem; they can also be quite painful. Essential oils such as cypress, geranium, helichrysum, lavender, and lemongrass can help speed healing while bringing relief from discomfort. Use an ice pack over a blend of cypress and lavender to constrict blood vessels right after a bruise occurs. For older bruises, my go-to is a blend of several oils that increase circulation so damaged tissue heals faster.

Helichrysum Neat Treatment

MAKES 1 TREATMENT

2 drops helichrysum essential oil

Apply the helichrysum essential oil directly to the bruised area, using a little more or less depending on the size of the site. Repeat two to three times daily or as needed.

TIP If you don't have helichrysum essential oil, you can treat a painful bruise by applying lavender neat instead.

Lavender-Cypress Salve

MAKES ABOUT 1 TEASPOON

1 teaspoon jojoba oil

4 drops lavender essential oil

3 drops cypress essential oil →

Lavender-Cypress Salve continued

1. In a small bottle with a tight-fitting lid and an orifice reducer, combine the jojoba oil with the lavender and cypress essential oils. Secure the lid and shake well to blend.
2. Apply 2 drops of the blend to a fresh bruise, using more if the painful area is large.
3. Cover the area with a soft cloth and apply an ice pack for 10 to 15 minutes. Repeat two to three times daily or as needed.

STORAGE Keep in a cool, dark place.

TIP This blend can help with dark under-eye circles, too. Apply just one drop under each eye before applying cosmetics and another just before bed.

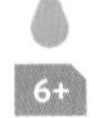

Healing Massage Oil

MAKES ABOUT 2 OUNCES

2 ounces jojoba oil

15 drops helichrysum essential oil

12 drops lavender essential oil

9 drops lemongrass essential oil

9 drops geranium essential oil

9 drops cypress essential oil

1. In a small bottle or jar with a tight-fitting lid, combine the jojoba oil with the helichrysum, lavender, lemongrass, geranium, and cypress essential oils. Secure the lid and shake well to blend.

2. Apply ½ teaspoon of the blend to the affected area and gently massage until the remedy is absorbed. Use more for larger areas. Repeat once or twice daily.

STORAGE Keep in a cool, dark place.

TIP Make a milder version of this oil to treat children under 6 years by omitting the geranium and lemongrass. Add an extra 3 drops of helichrysum, 2 drops of lavender, and 1 drop of cypress.

BURN

From the kitchen to campfires, minor burns can happen even when you think you're being careful, so it's always a good idea to keep a burn remedy handy. The essential oils in these remedies help stop the pain and promote faster healing, too. My steadfast remedy for little burns is lavender essential oil, applied neat. A neat treatment feels a bit cooler and prevents the momentary worsening of pain that often accompanies swabbing.

Eucalyptus–Tea Tree Spray

MAKES ABOUT 4 OUNCES

3 ounces alcohol-free witch hazel

1 ounce aloe vera gel

20 drops eucalyptus essential oil

20 drops tea tree essential oil →

Eucalyptus–Tea Tree Spray continued

1. In a small bottle with a fine-mist spray top, combine the witch hazel and aloe gel with the eucalyptus and tea tree essential oils and secure the top. Shake well before each use.
2. Apply a single spritz to the burn, and repeat the treatment two to three times daily.

STORAGE Keep in a cool, dark place.

TIP This spray is also ideal for treating sunburns. Apply it to the affected areas as often as needed to cool the sting.

Lavender Neat Treatment

MAKES 1 TREATMENT

1 or 2 drops lavender essential oil

1. Run cold water over the burn for 60 seconds (if possible) and then carefully pat dry the area *surrounding* the burn, taking care not to touch the burn itself.
2. Apply the lavender essential oil directly onto the burn. Repeat again in 20 to 30 minutes, then repeat two to three times daily.

TIP If you're out of lavender essential oil but have Roman chamomile on hand, give it a try. The healing effect may not be as pronounced, but chamomile can soothe pain and stop blistering.

Helichrysum Burn Salve

MAKES ABOUT 1 OUNCE

1 ounce aloe vera gel

20 drops helichrysum essential oil

1. In a small jar with a tight-fitting lid, combine the aloe gel with the helichrysum essential oil. Stir well with a thin utensil.
2. Apply a dime-size amount of the salve to the burn two to three times daily.

STORAGE Keep in a cool, dark place.

TIP For on-the-go healing, apply 1 drop of helichrysum neat, two to three times daily.

CHAPPED LIPS

Wind, salty seawater, and dry indoor air are just a few things that can cause chapped lips. The cracking and peeling is sometimes nothing more than a cosmetic problem, but when fissures develop, chapping can become painful. Helichrysum, frankincense, and Roman chamomile are a few of the most soothing essential oils to use for speedy healing of chapped lips. →

Chamomile-Frankincense Balm

MAKES ABOUT ½ OUNCE

1 tablespoon jojoba oil

3 drops frankincense essential oil

3 drops Roman chamomile essential oil

1. In a small glass tube with a tight-fitting lid and roller top, combine the jojoba oil with the frankincense and Roman chamomile essential oils. Secure the top and shake well to blend.
2. Apply liberally to your lips two to three times daily.

STORAGE Keep in a convenient place.

TIP If you don't have a tube with a roller top, you can use a small bottle with a tight-fitting lid and an orifice reducer instead. Use your finger to apply a drop or two to each of your lips.

Lavender-Helichrysum Lip Salve

MAKES ABOUT ½ OUNCE

1 tablespoon extra-virgin coconut oil, softened

6 drops helichrysum essential oil

4 drops lavender essential oil

1. In a small jar, combine the coconut oil with the helichrysum and lavender essential oils. Stir well with a thin utensil and allow the mixture to solidify.
2. Transfer the solid mixture to a lip balm jar.
3. Use your fingertip to apply the salve to your lips three to four times daily.

STORAGE Keep in a cool place; coconut oil melts at body temperature.

TIP If you prefer a liquid version of this salve, use jojoba oil instead of coconut and use a small glass tube with a roller top to apply.

CHICKEN POX

Chicken pox is caused by a highly contagious virus, and once your child gets it, there's nothing to do but keep him or her as comfortable as possible while the illness runs its course. It takes an average of 10 days from the time the first spots appear to the time all the blisters have dried and crusted over. Call your doctor immediately if constant vomiting, sensitivity to light, a severe headache, confusion, unusual sleepiness, breathing problems, or signs of skin infection occur.

Soothing Lavender Bath

MAKES 1 TREATMENT

1 cup baking soda

3 drops lavender essential oil

1. Draw a warm bath. Dissolve the baking soda in the water and then add the lavender essential oil.
2. Soak for at least 15 minutes. Towel off by gently patting dry. Repeat once or twice daily while discomfort persists.

TIP This bath can also help soothe some of the itching from a sunburn that's in the process of healing.

Chamomile-Eucalyptus Blend

MAKES ABOUT 4 OUNCES

4 ounces alcohol-free witch hazel

20 drops Roman chamomile essential oil

20 drops eucalyptus essential oil

1. In a small bottle with a tight-fitting lid and an orifice reducer, combine the witch hazel with the Roman chamomile and eucalyptus essential oils. Secure the lid and shake well to blend.
2. Apply 5 drops to a cotton ball and swab affected areas, using more if needed. Repeat the treatment two to three times daily.

STORAGE Keep in a convenient location if using frequently; otherwise, keep in a cool, dark place.

TIP In a pinch, use either tea tree or lavender essential oil neat by using a cotton swab to apply a drop or two to the affected area two to three times daily.

Lavender-Chamomile Calamine Lotion

MAKES ABOUT 4 OUNCES

1 (4-ounce) bottle calamine lotion

10 drops lavender essential oil

10 drops Roman chamomile essential oil

1. Remove the seal from the bottle of lotion. Add the lavender and Roman chamomile essential oils directly to the bottle. Secure the lid and shake well to blend.

2. Apply 1 or 2 teaspoons at a time, using just enough to cover all the pox with a thin layer of the lotion.

STORAGE Keep in a cool, dark place.

TIP If calamine lotion isn't available, you can use 4 ounces of aloe vera gel instead.

COLD

From coughing and stuffy sinuses to exhaustion and frustration, cold symptoms can make even the most beautiful day feel like a miserable one. Fortunately, you can ease some of your suffering by using essential oils that support your immune system. They can provide you with a good dose of relief while your body heals itself—minus the side effects that often accompany OTC remedies.

Decongestant Rub

MAKES ABOUT 2 OUNCES

2 ounces unscented body lotion
4 drops tea tree essential oil
2 drops lemon essential oil
2 drops thyme essential oil
2 drops rosemary essential oil

1. In a small jar with a tight-fitting lid, combine the body lotion with the tea tree, lemon, thyme, and rosemary essential oils. Stir well with a thin utensil. →

Decongestant Rub continued

2. Apply ½ teaspoon of the lotion to the chest and neck. Repeat two to three times daily.

STORAGE Keep in a cool, dark place.

TIP If you don't have unscented body lotion, use 2 ounces of your favorite carrier oil.

Lavender-Marjoram Bath Oil

MAKES ABOUT 4 OUNCES

4 ounces jojoba oil

20 drops lavender essential oil

20 drops marjoram essential oil

1. In a small bottle or jar with a tight-fitting lid, combine the jojoba oil with the lavender and marjoram essential oils. Secure the lid and shake well to blend.
2. Draw a hot bath and add ½ tablespoon of the oil blend. Remain in the tub for at least 15 minutes, relaxing and breathing deeply.

STORAGE Keep in a cool, dark place.

TIP If you don't have marjoram essential oil on hand, replace it with 10 drops of tea tree or 20 drops of eucalyptus.

Citrus-Eucalyptus Vapor

MAKES 1 TREATMENT

2 cups steaming hot (not boiling) water

2 drops lemon essential oil

2 drops sweet orange essential oil

4 drops eucalyptus essential oil

1. Pour the water into a shallow bowl and add the lemon, sweet orange, and eucalyptus essential oils.
2. Sitting comfortably in front of the bowl, drape a towel over your head and the bowl, creating a tent that concentrates the steam and vapors. Breathe deeply until the water cools and the vapors subside, emerging for cool air as needed. Repeat once or twice daily.

TIP As an alternative to the vapor tent for children under 12 years, diffuse the essential oils a few feet away from the activity area or in the child's bedroom. A vaporizer or humidifier is another option.

COLD SORE

Let's face it: cold sores aren't just uncomfortable; they can make you feel self-conscious, too. Essential oils can ease the itching and burning that accompany a cold sore, and they can help shorten its duration. The most effective ones have antiviral properties; geranium, juniper, tea tree, and lemongrass are some to consider. ➛

Geranium Compress

6+

MAKES 1 TREATMENT

1 drop geranium essential oil

1. Dampen a cotton ball with cool water and squeeze out the excess moisture. Apply the geranium essential oil to the cotton ball.
2. Press the cotton ball against your cold sore, leaving it in place for 30 seconds to 1 minute. Repeat twice daily until the cold sore has healed.

TIP Replace the geranium essential oil with lavender if treating a child under 6 years.

Lavender–Tea Tree Salve

MAKES ABOUT ½ OUNCE

1 tablespoon extra-virgin olive oil

5 drops tea tree essential oil

5 drops lavender essential oil

1. In a small jar with a tight-fitting lid, combine the olive oil with the tea tree and lavender essential oils. Secure the lid and shake well to blend.
2. Use a cotton swab to apply 1 drop of the mixture to the cold sore. Reapply three to four times daily while the cold sore is healing.

STORAGE Keep in a cool, dark place.

TIP Double the lavender and omit the tea tree if treating a child under 12 years.

COLIC

Colic means discomfort for your baby and sleepless nights for you. The cause of this condition, characterized by repeated bouts of crying in an otherwise healthy baby, is unknown; however, gas, overstimulation, and uncomfortable tummy muscles often play a role. Before using these gentle remedies to treat your baby's colic, be sure to have your pediatrician rule out any potential medical issues that may be contributing to the fussiness.

Lavender-Chamomile Vapor

MAKES 1 TREATMENT

Distilled or purified water

3 drops lavender essential oil

3 drops Roman chamomile essential oil

1. Following the manufacturer's instructions, add the called-for amount of water and the lavender and Roman chamomile essential oils to your humidifier or steam vaporizer.
2. Run the humidifier or vaporizer for 1 hour in the room where the baby is spending the most time. Repeat three to four times daily, or less often as needed.

TIP You can use a diffuser instead of a vaporizer or humidifier, but first dilute the essential oils 1:1 with a carrier oil before adding the blend to the diffuser; follow the manufacturer's instructions for use.

Soothing Tummy Massage

MAKES ABOUT 8 OUNCES

8 ounces sweet almond oil

8 drops lavender essential oil

8 drops geranium essential oil

8 drops Roman chamomile essential oil

1. In a small bottle or jar with a tight-fitting lid, combine the sweet almond oil with the lavender, geranium, and Roman chamomile essential oils. Secure the lid and shake well to blend.
2. Using your fingertips, apply 1 teaspoon of the blend to the baby's back and abdomen. Dress your baby and apply a warm (not hot) water bottle to the abdomen. Leave it in place for 10 or 15 minutes.

STORAGE Keep in a cool, dark place.

TIP Don't worry if you're missing the water bottle; it adds comfort and can help your baby relax, but it isn't absolutely essential to the treatment.

CONJUNCTIVITIS

The redness, swelling, and discomfort of conjunctivitis can affect one or both eyes. Though it typically resolves on its own, you can speed healing along with the careful use of essential oils, especially clary sage, which is also used to address issues such as tired or strained eyes. Its ability to reduce inflammation brings comfort, and its antibacterial properties can help prevent infection. Use great care with these remedies, ensuring that no essential oil comes into contact with eye tissue.

Clary Sage Eye Compress

MAKES 1 TREATMENT

½ cup warm water

2 drops clary sage essential oil

1. Pour the water into a shallow bowl and add the clary sage essential oil. Soak a soft cloth in the mixture and wring it out.
2. Fold the cloth and press it gently over the affected eye or eyes, keeping the eye(s) closed during the entire treatment. Leave it in place for 10 minutes. Repeat two to three times daily.

TIP For relief at times when a compress isn't practical, diffuse 2 or 3 drops of clary sage essential oil a few feet away from your face.

Chamomile Vapor

MAKES 1 TREATMENT

2 cups steaming hot (not boiling) water

2 drops Roman chamomile essential oil

1. Pour the water into a shallow bowl and add the Roman chamomile essential oil. Sit comfortably in front of the bowl and inhale the vapor while keeping your eyes open and blinking normally. →

Chamomile Vapor continued

2. Continue the treatment for 10 minutes or until the water stops steaming. Repeat two to three times daily.

TIP For relief at times when a vapor treatment isn't practical, diffuse 2 or 3 drops of Roman chamomile essential oil a few feet away from your face. For children under 2 years, dilute the essential oil 1:1 with carrier oil before adding it to the diffuser.

CONSTIPATION

Difficult or infrequent bowel movements lead to symptoms that range from mild discomfort to serious swelling and abdominal pain. Essential oils can bring comfort while helping move the digestive process along. If you've addressed any dietary causes of constipation and still suffer from it frequently, be sure to get a checkup from your doctor to rule out an underlying medical cause.

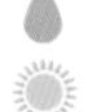

6+

Minty Rosemary-Lemon Abdominal Massage Oil

MAKES ABOUT 4 OUNCES

4 ounces jojoba oil

60 drops rosemary essential oil

40 drops lemon essential oil

20 drops peppermint essential oil

1. In a small bottle or jar with a tight-fitting lid, combine the jojoba oil with the rosemary, lemon, and peppermint essential oils. Secure the lid and shake well to blend.
2. About 2 hours after a meal, lie flat on your back with your knees drawn up. Apply 1 tablespoon of the blend to your abdomen and gently massage, making clockwise motions around your navel. Avoid making counterclockwise motions, as this can make constipation worse. Repeat two to three times daily.

STORAGE Keep in a cool, dark place.

TIP For children under 6 years, replace the peppermint with spearmint and use ½ tablespoon of massage oil for each treatment.

Ginger-Mandarin Aromatherapy

MAKES 1 TREATMENT

4 drops carrier oil

2 drops ginger essential oil

2 drops mandarin essential oil

1. In the palm of your hand, combine the carrier oil with the ginger and mandarin essential oils. Rub your hands together briefly and then rub the blend onto the soles of your feet or gently massage into your lower abdomen.

TIP If you'd like to try an alternative to the ginger essential oil, consider 2 drops of patchouli or cedarwood.

COUGH

Dry, persistent coughing may be caused by another condition or it can pop up unexpectedly with no other symptoms. To get relief, you can use essential oils on their own or alongside other cough-relieving remedies. Eucalyptus, thyme, and tea tree are excellent oils for this ailment, as they can settle the cough while addressing any allergens or irritants that might be contributing to it.

Soothing Eucalyptus Vapor

6+

MAKES 1 TREATMENT

4 drops eucalyptus essential oil

1. Prepare a steamy shower, then apply the eucalyptus essential oil to a washcloth.
2. Place the cloth in the shower at the end opposite the showerhead. Enjoy a long shower while breathing deeply.

TIP If you prefer bathing to showering, you can add the essential oil directly to a hot bath. For children under 6 years, use 4 drops of lavender, frankincense, or Roman chamomile essential oil instead of eucalyptus.

Chamomile-Frankincense Chest Rub

MAKES ABOUT 2 OUNCES

2 ounces unscented body lotion

16 drops Roman chamomile essential oil

12 drops frankincense essential oil

1. In a small jar with a tight-fitting lid, combine the body lotion with the Roman chamomile and frankincense essential oils. Stir well with a thin utensil.
2. Apply 1 teaspoon of the mixture to the chest and throat. Use ½ teaspoon for young children and a bit more than that for older children. Repeat two to three times daily.

STORAGE Keep in a cool, dark place.

TIP For a stronger blend that's suitable for adults and children over 6 years, add 12 drops of eucalyptus essential oil and replace the frankincense with 12 drops of thyme.

CRADLE CAP

Cradle cap can be a scary-looking condition, but it won't cause any discomfort or harm your baby if you get it under control before redness develops. If cracking or irritation is present, be sure to see your pediatrician to rule out infection. Mild essential oils such as frankincense, myrrh, and sandalwood can help loosen the scales, as can brushing with a soft-bristled baby brush.

Myrrh Massage Oil

MAKES ABOUT 1 OUNCE

1 ounce sweet almond oil

4 drops myrrh essential oil →

Myrrh Massage Oil continued

1. In a small bottle or jar with a tight-fitting lid, combine the sweet almond oil with the myrrh essential oil. Secure the lid and shake well to blend.
2. Apply ¼ teaspoon of the mixture to your baby's scalp, gently massaging the affected area. Leave the treatment in place for 15 minutes and then use a fine-toothed comb to remove flakes that have come off.
3. Wash the baby's head with mild soap and water, ensuring that you remove all of the oil. Repeat once daily.

STORAGE Keep in a cool, dark place.

TIP Use frankincense instead of myrrh if you prefer.

Lavender Scalp Spray

MAKES ABOUT 4 OUNCES

4 ounces distilled or purified water

6 drops lavender essential oil

1. In a small bottle with a fine-mist spray top, combine the water with the lavender essential oil and secure the top. Shake well before each use.
2. Apply a fine mist of spray to your baby's scalp after each bath and at bedtime.

STORAGE Keep in a cool, dark place.

TIP If you don't have a spray bottle, apply ¼ teaspoon of the mixture to a cotton ball and swab the baby's scalp.

CUT

Minor cuts can happen virtually anywhere—in the kitchen, on the playground, at work, and in a myriad of other places. Essential oils like lavender, tea tree, and eucalyptus are excellent first-aid remedies. They fight bacteria and help speed healing. Leave your cut or scrape exposed to air for a while after one of these treatments so that a scab can form. Yes, scabs might look disgusting, but they protect the skin and help it heal.

Frankincense-Helichrysum Salve

MAKES ABOUT 2 OUNCES

2 ounces aloe vera gel

10 drops frankincense essential oil

10 drops helichrysum essential oil

1. In a small jar with a tight-fitting lid, combine the aloe gel with the frankincense and helichrysum essential oils. Stir well with a thin utensil.
2. Apply a pea-size amount of the salve to the affected area, using a little more or less if needed. Repeat the treatment two to three times daily.

STORAGE Keep in a cool, dark place.

TIP If you don't have frankincense essential oil, you can use 10 drops of lavender instead.

Lavender Neat Treatment

MAKES 1 TREATMENT

4 drops lavender essential oil

1. Clean the affected area with soap and water. Rinse well and pat dry.
2. Apply the lavender essential oil directly onto the wound. You might need a bit more if you're treating a large area such as a skinned elbow or knee. Repeat twice daily.

TIP For adults and children over 6 years, you can use eucalyptus essential oil neat, if you prefer. It stops pain quickly and is fantastic for paper cuts.

First-Aid Antiseptic Spray

MAKES ABOUT 8 OUNCES

5 ounces aloe vera gel

3 ounces alcohol-free witch hazel

40 drops lavender essential oil

30 drops tea tree essential oil

10 drops myrrh essential oil

10 drops thyme essential oil

1. In a small bottle with a fine-mist spray top, combine the aloe gel and witch hazel with the lavender, tea tree, myrrh, and thyme essential oils and secure the top. Shake well before each use.
2. Clean the affected area and spray generously. Repeat two to three times daily.

STORAGE Keep in a cool, dark place.

TIP Make a similar remedy for children under 6 years by omitting the tea tree essential oil.

DANDRUFF

Flakes on our shoulders are something we all want to avoid, but even if others can't see it, the itchiness associated with dandruff can feel unbearable. Astringent essential oils like rosemary and lemon cut through the excess oil that contributes to the problem. At the same time, they contribute to soft, shiny hair. Be sure to use warm rather than hot water on your head. It will rinse effectively without contributing to the overdrying that can throw your scalp out of balance.

Lavender-Lemon Leave-In Conditioner

MAKES ABOUT 8 OUNCES

2 ounces unscented conditioner

6 ounces distilled or purified water

20 drops lavender essential oil

10 drops lemon essential oil

1. In a small bottle with a fine-mist spray top, combine the conditioner and water with the lavender and lemon essential oils and secure the top. Shake well before each use. ➛

Lavender-Lemon Leave-In Conditioner continued

2. Spritz your freshly washed hair five to six times, and then massage gently into your scalp.
3. Use a fine-toothed comb to remove any visible flakes and then allow your hair to dry naturally. Style as usual.

STORAGE Keep in a cool, dark place.

TIP For thick hair, use 3 ounces of conditioner to 5 ounces of water. For baby-fine hair, use 1 ounce of conditioner to 7 ounces of water.

Rosemary-Cedarwood Shampoo

MAKES ABOUT 8 OUNCES

7 ounces unscented shampoo

1 ounce alcohol-free witch hazel

20 drops rosemary essential oil

20 drops cedarwood essential oil

1. In a small squeeze bottle, combine the shampoo and witch hazel with the rosemary and cedarwood essential oils. Secure the top and shake well to blend.
2. Shampoo your hair with 1 teaspoon of shampoo, using a little more or less as needed. Repeat the treatment once daily.

STORAGE Keep this shampoo in the shower if you plan to use it all within 2 weeks; otherwise, keep in a cool, dark place.

TIP If you don't have rosemary and cedarwood, you can make this shampoo with equal amounts of lavender and tea tree essential oils instead.

6+

Healing Tea Tree Hair Mask

MAKES ABOUT 4 OUNCES

4 ounces jojoba oil

60 drops tea tree essential oil

30 drops lavender essential oil

1. In a small bottle or jar with a tight-fitting lid, combine the jojoba oil with the tea tree and lavender essential oils. Secure the lid and shake well to blend.
2. Wet your hair and apply 1 tablespoon of the mixture to your head, using your fingertips to massage your scalp gently. Leave the treatment in place for 15 minutes, then wash and condition your hair as usual. Repeat daily in cases of severe dandruff; use once or twice weekly as a preventive.

STORAGE Keep in a cool, dark place.

TIP For children under 6 years, omit the tea tree essential oil and double the drops of lavender.

DIAPER RASH

Despite your best efforts to keep your little one clean and dry, diaper rash can still develop. Essential oils work best in mild cases, and myrrh, frankincense, and lavender are three reliable ones to use for healing rashes. If the rash looks swollen or infected, or if areas are cracking or bleeding, be sure to see your pediatrician for a stronger remedy. →

Soothing Chamomile-Lavender Spray

MAKES ABOUT 4 OUNCES

2 ounces jojoba oil

2 ounces distilled or purified water

40 drops lavender essential oil

20 drops Roman chamomile essential oil

1. In a small bottle with a fine-mist spray top, combine the jojoba oil and water with the lavender and Roman chamomile essential oils and secure the top. Shake well before each use.
2. After each diaper change, wash and dry your baby as usual. Spritz the affected area three to four times, and allow to air dry before putting on a fresh diaper.

STORAGE Keep in a cool, dark place.

TIP Make a soothing balm by increasing the jojoba oil to 4 ounces and eliminating the water.

Protective Frankincense Ointment

MAKES ABOUT 1½ OUNCES

1 (1½-ounce) tube lanolin

20 drops frankincense essential oil

1. Melt the lanolin by dropping the tube in a cup of very hot water and allowing it to sit for about 10 minutes. Carefully open the tube and transfer the melted lanolin to a small jar with a tight-fitting lid.

2. Add the frankincense essential oil to the jar and stir to blend. Allow to cool completely, stirring every 5 minutes or so.
3. After each diaper change, wash and dry your baby as usual. Apply a thin layer of the ointment to the affected areas; a dab about half the size of a dime is probably a little more than enough. Repeat after every diaper change.

STORAGE Keep in a cool, dark place.

TIP This ointment is fantastic for chapped hands and cracked cuticles, too.

Frankincense and Myrrh Powder

MAKES ABOUT 8 OUNCES

1 cup non-GMO cornstarch

20 drops frankincense essential oil

20 drops myrrh essential oil

1. In a glass or stainless-steel sugar shaker, combine the cornstarch with the frankincense and myrrh essential oils. Secure the top and shake well from side to side to blend.
2. After each diaper change, wash and dry your baby's bum as usual.
3. Apply Soothing Chamomile-Lavender Spray (page 102) or Protective Frankincense Ointment (page 102) to the affected area. Then apply a few shakes of powder before putting on a fresh diaper. ➔

Frankincense and Myrrh Powder continued

STORAGE Keep in a convenient location if using frequently; otherwise, keep in a cool, dark place.

TIP If you like, you can replace the cornstarch with unscented, no-talc baby powder. You can also replace the frankincense and myrrh essential oils with your choice of lavender or chamomile, or a combination of both.

DIARRHEA

At home and on the road, diarrhea might crop up for a variety of reasons. Whether caused by a virus or bacteria or experienced as a side effect of antibiotics or another medication, it can leave you feeling uncomfortable and dehydrated. Soothing essential oils, including geranium, ginger, frankincense, and Roman chamomile, offer relief and support your digestive system while you get back on track. If a virus or bacteria is to blame, try thyme, tea tree, lemon, eucalyptus, or lavender.

Peppermint-Eucalyptus Massage Oil

MAKES ABOUT 1 OUNCE

1 ounce jojoba oil

20 drops peppermint essential oil

20 drops eucalyptus essential oil

1. In a small bottle or jar with a tight-fitting lid, combine the jojoba oil with the peppermint and eucalyptus essential oils. Secure the lid and shake well to blend.

2. Apply 1 teaspoon of the blend to your lower abdomen, gently massaging until absorbed. Repeat two to three times daily.

STORAGE Keep in a cool, dark place.

TIP For children under 6 years, replace the peppermint and eucalyptus essential oils with an equal amount of Roman chamomile and spearmint.

Aromatherapy Bath Blend

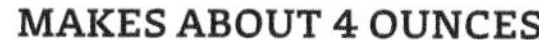

MAKES ABOUT 4 OUNCES

4 ounces jojoba oil
16 drops peppermint essential oil
16 drops lavender essential oil
16 drops eucalyptus essential oil
16 drops geranium essential oil
16 drops Roman chamomile essential oil

1. In a small bottle or jar with a tight-fitting lid, combine the jojoba oil with the peppermint, lavender, eucalyptus, geranium, and Roman chamomile essential oils. Secure the lid and shake well to blend.
2. Draw a hot bath and add 1 tablespoon of the blend to the bathtub. Soak for at least 15 minutes. Repeat once daily.

STORAGE Keep in a cool, dark place.

TIP This synergistic blend also works well for abdominal massage. To use, massage 1 teaspoon into your lower abdomen once or twice daily.

DRY SKIN

More than just a cosmetic issue, dry skin can bring itchiness and discomfort. Anti-inflammatory essential oils, including frankincense, geranium, and myrrh, help soothe irritation while promoting healing. You can help the process along by drinking plenty of water and opting for warm baths and showers over hot ones.

Sweet Orange–Ylang-Ylang Salve

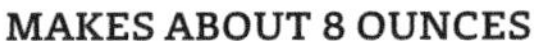

MAKES ABOUT 8 OUNCES

8 ounces extra-virgin coconut oil, softened

30 drops sweet orange essential oil

20 drops ylang-ylang essential oil

1. In a small jar with a tight-fitting lid, combine the coconut oil with the sweet orange and ylang-ylang essential oils. Stir well with a thin utensil.
2. Apply ¼ teaspoon of the blend to areas of dry skin, using a little more or less to cover the affected areas. Repeat at least once daily.

STORAGE Keep in a cool, dark place.

TIP If you plan to spend time in the sun, replace the sweet orange essential oil with an equal amount of geranium or myrrh.

Hydrating Facial Gel

MAKES ABOUT 4 OUNCES

4 ounces aloe vera gel

24 drops frankincense essential oil

12 drops geranium essential oil

1. In a small jar with a tight-fitting lid, combine the aloe gel with the frankincense and geranium essential oils. Stir well with a thin utensil.
2. Apply ¼ teaspoon of the gel to your freshly washed face each morning and evening. Use a little more if your skin is very thirsty.

STORAGE Keep in a cool, dark place.

TIP You can use this light, refreshing gel all over your body if you like. Omit the geranium for children under 6 years.

Frankincense and Myrrh Lotion

MAKES ABOUT 8 OUNCES

8 ounces unscented body lotion

32 drops frankincense essential oil

16 drops myrrh essential oil

1. In a small jar with a tight-fitting lid, combine the body lotion with the frankincense and myrrh essential oils. Stir well with a thin utensil.
2. Apply a dime-size amount of the lotion to each area of dry skin. Use a bit more if your skin is drinking up the lotion quickly. Reapply two to three times daily. →

Frankincense and Myrrh Lotion continued

STORAGE Keep in a cool, dark place.

TIP For a richer blend suitable for massage use, add 2 tablespoons of jojoba oil.

EAR INFECTION

Minor ear infections often respond well to treatment with essential oils, especially when you start treatment at the first sign of a problem. Since bacteria is to blame for this condition, the essential oils to use are those with strong antibacterial action. Tea tree, lavender, eucalyptus, and rosemary are good choices. Treatments that include oregano or clove essential oil will help ease discomfort. Call a doctor if pain becomes severe.

Oregano Poultice

MAKES 1 TREATMENT

2 drops carrier oil

2 drops oregano essential oil

1. Apply the carrier oil and the oregano essential oil to a cotton ball. Tuck the cotton ball into the affected ear.
2. Lie down with the painful ear pointing toward the ceiling. Leave it in place for 15 to 30 minutes. Repeat twice daily.

TIP If you are treating someone 6 years or older and don't have oregano, you can use clove instead, placing just 1 drop of clove essential oil and 2 drops of carrier oil onto the cotton ball.

Eucalyptus-Rosemary Aromatherapy

MAKES 1 TREATMENT

2 drops carrier oil

1 drop eucalyptus essential oil

1 drop rosemary essential oil

1. Apply the carrier oil to the area behind the ear, tracing a line beneath the outer corner of the jaw and extending it diagonally down the side of the neck all the way to the junction of the collarbones and the neck.
2. Apply the eucalyptus essential oil on top of the carrier oil, following the same path. Wait two minutes and then apply the rosemary essential oil, following the same path again. Repeat twice daily.

TIP For children under 6 years, replace the eucalyptus essential oil with lavender.

EARACHE

Whether an earache happens on its own or is accompanied by cold symptoms such as a sore throat and the sniffles, the discomfort is usually the same. A combination of heat and lavender essential oil is my go-to remedy for stopping earaches in their tracks; other oils to try include tea tree, lavender, thyme, and Roman chamomile. ➔

Chamomile–Tea Tree Aromatherapy

MAKES 1 TREATMENT

2 drops carrier oil

1 drop Roman chamomile essential oil

1 drop tea tree essential oil

In the palm of your hand, combine the carrier oil with the Roman chamomile and tea tree essential oils, mixing briefly with your fingertips. Gently apply the blend to the surface of the outer ear, the area behind the ear, and the jawline. Repeat twice daily.

TIP For children under 6 years, replace the tea tree essential oil with lavender and follow the same protocol.

Lavender-Thyme Poultice

MAKES 1 TREATMENT

2 drops carrier oil

1 drop lavender essential oil

1 drop thyme essential oil

1. Apply the carrier oil and the lavender and thyme essential oils to a cotton ball. Tuck the cotton ball into the affected ear.
2. Lie down with the painful ear pointing toward the ceiling, cover the side of your face with a soft cloth, then apply a hot water bottle or heat pack. Leave it in place for at least 15 minutes. Repeat two to three times daily.

TIP If you don't have thyme essential oil, try this remedy with 2 drops of lavender instead.

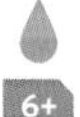

6+

Minty Lavender–Tea Tree Massage Oil

MAKES ABOUT 1 OUNCE

1 ounce carrier oil

30 drops peppermint essential oil

10 drops lavender essential oil

1. In a small bottle with a tight-fitting lid and an orifice reducer, combine the carrier oil with the peppermint and lavender essential oils. Secure the lid and shake well to blend.
2. Apply 3 drops to your fingertips and massage into the soft tissue surrounding the affected ear, using more if needed. Repeat two to three times daily.

STORAGE Keep in a cool, dark place.

TIP Treat children under 6 years by replacing the peppermint with spearmint.

ECZEMA

It's not easy to live with red, itchy, scaly skin or the swelling and inflammation that often accompany eczema. Because there are many contributing factors, including diet, you may have some sleuthing to do to get to the underlying cause of the problem. Meanwhile, soothing essential oils can bring relief quickly while helping skin heal. Use a moisturizing remedy for dry areas and a salt spray for weeping eczema. ➔

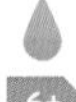

Peppermint-Juniper Sea Spray

6+

MAKES ABOUT 8 OUNCES

1 cup distilled or purified water

1 tablespoon fine sea salt

⅛ teaspoon Epsom salt

6 drops juniper essential oil

3 drops peppermint essential oil

1. In a small bottle with a fine-mist spray top, combine the water, sea salt, and Epsom salt with the juniper and peppermint essential oils. Secure the top and shake well to dissolve the salts.
2. Apply a single spritz to each affected area, blotting up any excess with a cotton pad. Repeat once or twice daily.

STORAGE Keep in a cool, dark place.

TIP For children under 6 years, replace the juniper and peppermint essential oils with 3 drops of spearmint and 6 drops of lavender.

Bergamot-Helichrysum Bath Oil

MAKES ABOUT 4 OUNCES

4 ounces carrier oil

20 drops bergamot essential oil

20 drops helichrysum essential oil

1. In a small bottle or jar with a tight-fitting lid, combine the carrier oil with the bergamot and helichrysum essential oils. Secure the lid and shake well to blend.

2. Draw a warm (not hot) bath, and add 1 tablespoon of the blend to the water. Spend at least 15 minutes soaking. Repeat every two days, or more frequently if desired.

STORAGE Keep in a cool, dark place.

TIP If you plan to spend time in the sun, replace the bergamot essential oil with geranium.

Geranium Aromatherapy

MAKES ABOUT 4 OUNCES

4 ounces extra-virgin coconut oil, softened

24 drops geranium essential oil

1. In a small jar with a tight-fitting lid, combine the coconut oil with the geranium essential oil. Secure the lid and shake well to blend.
2. Apply a dime-size amount of the blend to affected areas, using very light pressure to rub it in. You may need to use a bit more for large areas and a bit less for small areas. Repeat two to three times daily.

STORAGE Keep in a cool, dark place.

TIP For children under 6 years, replace the geranium essential oil with lavender.

EXHAUSTION

In today's busy world, the list of potential causes of exhaustion is endless. A good night's sleep is vital, but if that's not possible right away, energizing essential oils like lemon, grapefruit, and mandarin can provide the stimulation you need to get through tough times. When it's time to relax, other oils can ease tension and help you settle down.

Relaxing Downtime Diffusion

MAKES ABOUT ½ OUNCE

1 teaspoon patchouli essential oil

1 teaspoon frankincense essential oil

1 teaspoon myrrh essential oil

1. In a small bottle with a tight-fitting lid and an orifice reducer, combine the patchouli, frankincense, and myrrh essential oils. Secure the lid and shake well to blend.
2. Following the manufacturer's instructions, add 2 or 3 drops of the blend to your diffuser. Run the diffuser while you are relaxing. Repeat as often as you'd like.

STORAGE Keep in a cool, dark place.

TIP When measuring out essential oil in teaspoons, it helps to remove the orifice reducer from the bottle. You can also add 3 or 4 drops of this blend to a warm bath or place 1 drop on your pillowcase at bedtime.

Energizing Aromatic Spray

MAKES ABOUT 8 OUNCES

8 ounces distilled or purified water

32 drops mandarin essential oil

16 drops lemon essential oil

16 drops grapefruit essential oil

1. In a small bottle with a fine-mist spray top, combine the water with the mandarin, lemon, and grapefruit essential oils and secure the top. Shake well before each use.
2. Spritz your office chair, your clothing, or the interior of your car as often as you like.

STORAGE Keep in a cool, dark place.

TIP Create an energizing blend for your diffuser by eliminating the water and combining the mandarin, lemon, and grapefruit essential oils in a small bottle with a tight-fitting lid and an orifice reducer. Secure the lid and shake well to blend. Diffuse 2 or 3 drops in spaces where you spend time.

Lavender-Lemongrass Bath Blend

MAKES ABOUT 4 OUNCES

4 ounces carrier oil

20 drops lavender essential oil

10 drops lemongrass essential oil

1. In a small bottle or jar with a tight-fitting lid, combine the carrier oil with the lavender and lemongrass essential oils. Secure the lid and shake well to blend. ➛

Lavender-Lemongrass Bath Blend continued

2. Draw a hot bath and add 1 tablespoon of the blend to the water. Spend at least 15 minutes soaking. Repeat as often as you like.

STORAGE Keep in a cool, dark place.

TIP If you don't have time for a bath, you can diffuse a few drops of this blend or apply a drop each to your inner wrists, neck, and temples. If you don't have lemongrass essential oil, you can make a relaxing blend with an equal amount of Roman chamomile or rosemary, or double the amount of lavender for a simpler bath oil.

FEVER

Fever is the body's natural defense against infection. Febrifuge essential oils such as lemon and ginger can help bring down a fever, and cooling oils like spearmint and peppermint can help you feel more comfortable while you recover. When you are running a fever, remember to stay hydrated and rest. If a fever becomes dangerously high, seek medical attention.

Peppermint Neat Treatment

MAKES 1 TREATMENT

4 drops peppermint essential oil

Apply 1 drop of peppermint essential oil to each of your temples, and apply the other 2 drops to the nape of your neck.

TIP Make this treatment for children under 6 years by substituting spearmint essential oil, diluting it 1:1 with carrier oil, and applying as described.

Lemon-Ginger Compress

MAKES 1 TREATMENT

4 ounces water

4 ounces ice

8 drops ginger essential oil

4 drops lemon essential oil

1. Pour the water and ice into a shallow bowl and add the ginger and lemon essential oils. Dip a soft cloth into the bowl and wring out the excess liquid.
2. Lay the cloth across your forehead. Refresh it with more liquid when it warms, and repeat the process for at least 15 minutes.

TIP Make a cooling spray by eliminating the ice and combining the water with the ginger and lemon essential oils in a small bottle with a fine-mist spray top, and securing the lid. Shake well before each use. Spritz it onto your skin to help cool a fever or provide refreshment in hot weather, or enjoy it as a room spray.

Cooling Lavender-Spearmint Bath

MAKES 1 TREATMENT

6 drops lavender essential oil

6 drops spearmint essential oil

Draw a lukewarm bath and add the lavender and spearmint essential oils. Soak for at least 15 minutes. →

Cooling Lavender-Spearmint Bath continued

TIP Make a cooling massage blend by adding the lavender and spearmint essential oils to 1 tablespoon of carrier oil. To use, apply 4 drops to the back of your neck and massage into your hairline.

FLATULENCE

That cringe-worthy moment that accompanies flatulence in a public place is sometimes worse than the physical discomfort and bloating that often come with it. Peppermint, spearmint, and other digestive essential oils can help calm internal turbulence and provide comfort. Drink a hot cup of peppermint or chamomile tea to help speed relief.

Roman Chamomile Aromatherapy

MAKES 1 TREATMENT

6 drops carrier oil

6 drops Roman chamomile essential oil

In the palm of your hand, combine the carrier oil with the Roman chamomile essential oil. Rub your hands together briefly and then apply the blend to your inner wrists, neck, and temples.

TIP This remedy can also be helpful for treating insomnia. If you prefer, you can omit the carrier oil and diffuse the Roman chamomile essential oil in the space where you are spending the most time.

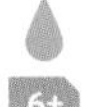
6+

Peppermint Massage Oil

MAKES ABOUT 1 OUNCE

2 tablespoons jojoba oil

30 drops peppermint essential oil

1. In a small bottle or jar with a tight-fitting lid, combine the jojoba oil with the peppermint essential oil. Secure the lid and shake well to blend.
2. Massage ½ teaspoon of the blend into the abdominal area two to three times daily.

STORAGE Keep in a cool, dark place.

TIP For children under 6 years, use ginger or spearmint instead of peppermint essential oil. For anyone 6 years or older, you can also use eucalyptus essential oil to combat flatulence.

FLU

A variety of viruses can cause different types of influenza. While essential oils don't cure the problem, they can help fight symptoms including coughing, body aches, exhaustion, and fever. Antiviral and antibacterial oils such as tea tree, eucalyptus, lavender, thyme, and clove are among the best for dealing with uncomfortable symptoms while giving your immune system a boost. →

Eucalyptus Room Spray

MAKES ABOUT 4 OUNCES

4 ounces distilled or purified water

25 drops eucalyptus essential oil

1. In a small bottle with a fine-mist spray top, combine the water with the eucalyptus essential oil and secure the top. Shake well before each use.
2. Spritz three to four times into the air and breathe deeply. Repeat every one to two hours.

STORAGE Keep in a cool, dark place.

TIP If you like, you can diffuse eucalyptus essential oil instead of spraying it. Use 2 or 3 drops at a time in your diffuser.

Relaxing Bath Salts

MAKES ABOUT 16 OUNCES

2 cups Epsom salt

10 drops cypress essential oil

10 drops lemon essential oil

5 drops tea tree essential oil

1. In a quart jar with a tight-fitting lid, combine the salt with the cypress, lemon, and tea tree essential oils. Secure the lid and shake well to blend.
2. Draw a warm bath. Add ½ cup of the bath salts and allow them to dissolve. Soak for 15 to 30 minutes. Repeat once or twice daily while recovering.

STORAGE Keep in a cool, dark place.

TIP These bath salts are ideal for treating cold symptoms, too. For children under 6 years, replace the tea tree essential oil with 10 drops of lavender.

Comforting Ginger-Clove Vapor

MAKES 1 TREATMENT

2 cups steaming hot (not boiling) water

2 drops ginger essential oil

1 drop clove essential oil

1. Pour the water into a shallow bowl and add the ginger and clove essential oils.
2. Sitting comfortably in front of the bowl, breathe deeply until the water cools and the vapors subside. Repeat once or twice daily.

TIP Resist the temptation to use a towel to create a tent when using this treatment; clove releases very strong vapors.

FROSTBITE

When skin freezes due to overexposure to frigid temperatures, frostbite can occur. Essential oils can help in minor cases of frostbite, increasing circulation to the injured area and mitigating damage to tissue and nerves. Skip the essential oils and seek emergency medical treatment for serious cases of frostbite. →

Lavender Neat Treatment

MAKES 1 TREATMENT

1 drop lavender essential oil

1. Gradually rewarm the affected area.
2. Apply the lavender essential oil directly to the affected area. Gently massage it in, adding another drop or two for larger areas.

TIP If you like, you can rewarm the whole body in a bath that contains 6 drops of lavender oil. Focus on massaging mild frostbite with the neat essential oil while relaxing in the bath.

Geranium-Clove Massage Oil

MAKES 1 TREATMENT

1 teaspoon carrier oil

5 drops geranium essential oil

2 drops clove essential oil

1. Gradually rewarm the affected area.
2. In the palm of your hand, combine the carrier oil with the geranium and clove essential oils. Rub your hands together briefly and then gently apply the blend to the affected areas.

TIP For children under 6 years, replace the geranium and clove with 7 drops of lavender essential oil.

HAND-FOOT-MOUTH DISEASE

Hand-foot-mouth disease is caused by a nasty virus that's notoriously difficult to eradicate. The symptoms are easy to spot: fever, itching, and painful blisters that cover the hands and feet and pop up inside the mouth, and sometimes progress to the face, knees, elbows, and genital area. Essential oils don't stop the blisters from developing, but they can help reduce pain and itching.

Chamomile-Cypress Lotion

MAKES ABOUT 4 OUNCES

4 ounces calamine lotion

10 drops Roman chamomile essential oil

8 drops cypress essential oil

1. In a small jar with a tight-fitting lid, combine the calamine lotion with the Roman chamomile and cypress essential oils. Stir well with a thin utensil.
2. Apply just enough of the mixture to cover the affected areas (excluding blisters in the mouth) with a thin layer. Repeat every three to four hours or as needed.

STORAGE Keep in a cool, dark place.

TIP If you don't have cypress essential oil, you can use 6 drops of lavender instead.

Soothing Lavender-Oatmeal Bath

MAKES 1 TREATMENT

1 single-use packet unscented oatmeal bath powder

10 drops lavender essential oil

1. Draw a warm bath and add the oatmeal powder. Stir it in with your hand, breaking up any lumps.
2. Add the lavender essential oil and then soak until the water cools. Pat dry and dress comfortably.

TIP This bath works well for a variety of skin conditions ranging from chicken pox to sunburn, and is suitable for people of all ages.

HAY FEVER

Sneezing; itchy, watery eyes; and a runny nose are signs that seasonal allergies are at work. Tea tree, eucalyptus, and niaouli are some of the best essential oils for relieving these symptoms, as are others with antihistamine properties. Besides diffusing these oils and using them in room sprays, you can make your home a sanctuary from seasonal allergens by keeping air filters clean, keeping windows and doors closed, and changing into fresh clothing as soon as you come in from outside.

Peppermint–Tea Tree Massage Oil

MAKES ABOUT 2 OUNCES

2 ounces carrier oil

20 drops peppermint essential oil

10 drops tea tree essential oil

1. In a small bottle or jar with a tight-fitting lid, combine the carrier oil with the peppermint and tea tree essential oils. Secure the lid and shake well to blend.
2. Apply 5 to 10 drops of the blend to your upper chest. Repeat two to three times daily or less often as needed.

STORAGE Keep in a cool, dark place.

TIP Prepare this remedy for children under 6 years by replacing the peppermint and tea tree essential oils with 30 drops of spearmint essential oil.

Niaouli Aromatherapy for Hay Fever

MAKES 1 TREATMENT

2 drops niaouli essential oil

1. On a handkerchief or other small cloth, apply 2 drops of niaouli essential oil. Hold the cloth 1 to 2 inches from your face and breathe deeply.
2. Continue the treatment for one to two minutes. Repeat every two to three hours.

TIP Ease breathing at night by placing two drops of niaouli essential oil on your pillowcase or diffusing it in your bedroom.

Tea Tree and Eucalyptus Diffusion

MAKES 1 TREATMENT

1 drop tea tree essential oil

2 drops eucalyptus essential oil

Following the manufacturer's instructions, add the tea tree and eucalyptus essential oils to your diffuser. Run the diffuser nearby. Repeat every two to three hours or as needed.

TIP This blend is fantastic for vapor therapy, too. Use it in a humidifier or vaporizer, or add the tea tree and eucalyptus essential oils to your bath.

HEADACHE

Even mild headaches can make everyday tasks seem insurmountable. Inflammation, tension, sinus congestion, and even bad lighting are a few of the many factors that contribute to head pain. Luckily, essential oils work quickly, and they may even keep you from reaching for OTC remedies. While simply inhaling essential oils can help ease minor pain, topical application is the most effective way to beat a tough headache. Lavender, peppermint, eucalyptus, and grapefruit are among the best essential oils to keep on hand for emergency relief.

Triple Essential Oil Diffusion

MAKES 1 TREATMENT

2 drops spearmint essential oil

1 drop lavender essential oil

1 drop rosemary essential oil

Following the manufacturer's instructions, add the spearmint, lavender, and rosemary essential oils to your diffuser. Run the diffuser nearby. Repeat every two to three hours or as needed.

TIP You can also create a blend by combining the spearmint, lavender, and rosemary essential oils with 1 tablespoon of carrier oil. Massage it into your neck and shoulders.

Grapefruit Massage Oil

MAKES ABOUT 4 OUNCES

4 ounces jojoba oil

20 drops grapefruit essential oil

1. In a small bottle with a tight-fitting lid, combine the jojoba oil and grapefruit essential oil. Secure the lid and shake well to blend.
2. Massage ¼ teaspoon of the blend into the back of your neck. Repeat every three to four hours or as needed.

STORAGE Keep in a cool, dark place.

TIP This blend is a good one for stress relief. You can use it to massage your hands, arms, shoulders, and neck, or put a tablespoon of the blend into a warm, relaxing bath.

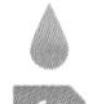

Peppermint Neat Treatment

MAKES 1 TREATMENT

2 drops peppermint essential oil

Apply 1 drop of peppermint essential oil to each of your temples. Or apply the essential oil to the head or neck where you feel pain most acutely.

TIP If treating a child under 6 years, replace the peppermint essential oil with spearmint.

Minty Lavender-Eucalyptus Balm for Sinus Headaches

MAKES ABOUT 1 OUNCE

1 ounce carrier oil

12 drops peppermint essential oil

12 drops lavender essential oil

8 drops eucalyptus essential oil

1. In a small bottle with a tight-fitting lid and an orifice reducer, combine the carrier oil with the peppermint, lavender, and eucalyptus essential oils. Secure the lid and shake well to blend.
2. Apply 1 or 2 drops of the blend onto your cheekbones, forehead, and temples and massage gently. Repeat every two to three hours or as needed.

STORAGE Keep in a cool, dark place.

TIP If treating a child under 6 years, omit the eucalyptus essential oil and replace the peppermint with spearmint.

HEARTBURN

An oversize portion of hot wings or a heaping serving of lasagna can lead to heartburn, which happens when acid escapes from your stomach and travels up toward your throat. While eating certain foods and frequent overeating in general are contributors to be aware of, other causes include stress, pregnancy, and being overweight. Essential oils such as marjoram, mandarin, lemon, and ginger support healthy digestion and can bring rapid relief while helping your body rid itself of toxins faster.

Marjoram Massage Oil

MAKES ABOUT 4 OUNCES

4 ounces jojoba oil

16 drops marjoram essential oil

1. In a small bottle or jar with a tight-fitting lid, combine the jojoba oil with the marjoram essential oil. Secure the lid and shake well to blend.
2. Apply ½ teaspoon of the blend to the chest and upper abdomen, massaging gently. Repeat every two to three hours or as needed.

STORAGE Keep in a cool, dark place.

TIP If you don't have marjoram, you can make the blend with peppermint or spearmint essential oil instead.

Peppermint-Ginger Salve

MAKES ABOUT 4 OUNCES

4 ounces aloe vera gel

30 drops peppermint essential oil

20 drops ginger essential oil

1. In a small jar with a tight-fitting lid, combine the aloe gel with the peppermint and ginger essential oils. Stir well with a thin utensil.
2. Apply ½ teaspoon of the salve to your upper abdomen, using a little more or less if needed. Repeat as often as needed.

STORAGE Keep in a cool, dark place.

TIP This salve is good for indigestion and upset stomachs, too. If treating a child under 6 years, replace the peppermint with spearmint essential oil.

Peppermint Neat Treatment

MAKES 1 TREATMENT

6 to 8 drops peppermint essential oil

1. Apply 3 or 4 drops of peppermint essential oil directly to the sole of each foot.
2. Lie down on your left side and relax while the essential oil absorbs. Repeat every two to three hours or as needed.

TIP Treat children under 6 years by replacing the peppermint with spearmint or marjoram essential oil.

HEAT RASH

Hot temperatures and high humidity can lead to painful, itchy heat rash, also known as summer rash or prickly heat. Anti-inflammatory essential oils bring rapid relief from the swelling, and those with analgesic properties can help with pain. You can speed healing by exposing the affected area to air, taking cool baths, and wearing loose, breathable clothing.

Chamomile-Lavender Spray

MAKES ABOUT 4 OUNCES

3 ounces alcohol-free witch hazel

1 ounce aloe vera gel

12 drops lavender essential oil

8 drops Roman chamomile essential oil

1. In a small bottle with a fine-mist spray top, combine the witch hazel and aloe gel with the lavender and Roman chamomile essential oils. Secure the top and shake well to blend.
2. Spritz each affected area once, and allow it to air dry before dressing. Repeat every two to three hours or as often as needed.

STORAGE Keep in a cool, dark place.

TIP For a stronger spray suitable for children over 6 years, add 12 drops of tea tree essential oil to the blend.

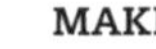

Lavender-Eucalyptus Soak

MAKES 1 TREATMENT

½ cup baking soda

8 drops lavender essential oil

4 drops eucalyptus essential oil

1. Draw a cool bath. Dissolve the baking soda in the water and add the lavender and eucalyptus essential oils.
2. Spend at least 15 minutes soaking. When you emerge, towel off by gently patting yourself dry. Ensure that no moisture remains on the affected areas. Repeat once or twice daily.

TIP Prepare a bath blend ahead of time by mixing the baking soda and lavender and eucalyptus essential oils together and then storing the mixture in a tightly sealed container. For children under 6 years, replace the eucalyptus with chamomile essential oil.

HEMORRHOIDS

When veins in the rectal region are subjected to excessive strain, the resulting inflammation leads to itching, pain, and swelling. While this problem isn't one that people usually talk about, it's actually quite common. Sufferers include pregnant women, people who are overweight, and those who are frequently constipated. Anti-inflammatory essential oils can help shrink swollen tissue and bring relief from discomfort, often just as quickly as OTC remedies.

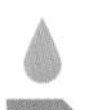

Tea Tree Salve

MAKES ABOUT 4 OUNCES

4 ounces lanolin

1 teaspoon tea tree essential oil

1. Melt the lanolin by dropping the tube into a cup of very hot water and allowing it to sit for about 10 minutes.
2. Carefully open the tube and transfer the melted lanolin to a small jar with a tight-fitting lid. Add the tea tree essential oil and stir to blend, using a thin utensil. Allow to cool completely, stirring every 5 minutes or so.
3. Using a cotton pad, apply ⅛ teaspoon of the salve to the rectal area. Repeat in the morning and evening as well as after each bowel movement.

STORAGE Keep in a cool, dark place.

TIP If treating a child under 6 years, replace the tea tree essential oil with myrrh.

Cooling Cypress Pads

MAKES 16 TREATMENTS

1 ounce alcohol-free witch hazel

16 drops cypress essential oil

16 cotton cosmetic pads

1. In a small jar with a tight-fitting lid, combine the witch hazel and cypress essential oil, then add the pads to the solution. ➛

Cooling Cypress Pads continued

2. Close the jar and invert it to allow the pads to soak up the solution.
3. Use a pad to gently swab the rectal area. Repeat two to three times daily, or more frequently if needed.

STORAGE Keep in a cool, dark place.

TIP If you are pregnant, replace the cypress essential oil with tea tree.

HICCUPS

Hiccups seem to pop up out of nowhere. In case you're wondering, they're caused by involuntary diaphragm contractions that pull air into your throat. To combat this annoying occurrence, turn to antispasmodic essential oils. They offer quick relief by encouraging your diaphragm to relax.

Mandarin Aromatherapy

MAKES 1 TREATMENT

3 drops mandarin essential oil

Apply the mandarin essential oil to a cotton ball or cloth and hold it 6 inches from your nose. Breathe deeply until the hiccups subside.

TIP You can substitute mandarin with Roman chamomile essential oil.

Chamomile-Ginger Inhaler

MAKES 1 TREATMENT

3 drops chamomile essential oil

2 drops ginger essential oil

1 paper lunch bag

1. Apply the chamomile and ginger essential oils to a cotton ball and then drop the cotton ball into the paper bag.
2. Cover your nose and mouth with the bag's opening, and take deep breaths until the hiccups subside.

TIP If you don't have chamomile and ginger essential oil, you can make this treatment with your choice of 5 drops of peppermint or spearmint.

Spearmint Abdominal Massage Oil

MAKES 1 TREATMENT

3 drops carrier oil

3 drops spearmint essential oil

1. In the palm of your hand, combine the carrier oil with the spearmint essential oil. Rub your hands together briefly and then gently massage the blend into your upper abdomen, focusing on the area just below your sternum.
2. Take deep, calming breaths until the hiccups subside.

TIP If an abdominal massage isn't practical, apply the spearmint essential oil to a cotton ball or a piece of cloth and hold it within a few inches of your nose while taking deep breaths.

HIVES

Stress, skin irritation, and allergies are some of the things that can cause a bad case of itchy red hives. Essential oils help put a stop to the symptoms while easing stress. Gentle topical applications work best for hives, but if you're in a situation where using them is impractical, try aromatherapy. Relief won't happen as quickly, but you'll still be targeting stress, allergies, and inflammation.

Triple Aromatherapy Gel

MAKES ABOUT 4 OUNCES

4 ounces aloe vera gel

10 drops cypress essential oil

10 drops lavender essential oil

10 drops Roman chamomile essential oil

1. In a small jar with a tight-fitting lid, combine the aloe gel with the cypress, lavender, and Roman chamomile essential oils. Stir well with a thin utensil.
2. Bathe or shower and pat dry. Apply ½ teaspoon of the gel in a thin layer, focusing on the affected area, using more or less as needed. After the gel dries, dress in loose, breathable clothing.

STORAGE Keep in a cool, dark place or store in the refrigerator for a cooling sensation with each use.

TIP This gel can also help you relax at bedtime. Just warm ½ teaspoon in your hands and apply it to your inner wrists, neck, and temples.

Healing Myrrh Bath

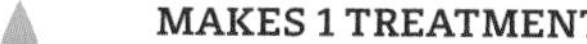

MAKES 1 TREATMENT

1 single-use packet unscented oatmeal bath powder

10 drops myrrh essential oil

1. Draw a lukewarm bath and add the oatmeal powder. Stir it in with your hand, breaking up any lumps, then add the myrrh essential oil.
2. Soak until the water cools. Pat yourself completely dry and dress in loose, breathable clothing.

TIP If you don't have myrrh essential oil, replace it with a blend of 10 drops of lavender and 5 drops of chamomile. For children over 6 years and adults, add 5 drops of peppermint essential oil.

HOT FLASHES

Low estrogen leads to a variety of uncomfortable symptoms, including unbearable hot flashes. Instead of reaching for a controversial prescription, consider treating your hot flashes naturally with essential oils. Cooling oils such as peppermint and spearmint bring immediate relief, and others, especially clary sage essential oil, contain plant estrogens that can help you manage your symptoms. →

Clary Sage Temple Massage Oil

MAKES ABOUT ⅓ OUNCE

2 teaspoons carrier oil

36 drops clary sage essential oil

1. In a small bottle with a tight-fitting lid and an orifice reducer, combine the carrier oil with the clary sage essential oil. Secure the lid and shake well to blend.
2. Apply 1 drop of the blend to each of your temples whenever you feel a hot flash coming on and/or apply 1 drop to the sole of each foot after your daily bath or shower, to reduce the occurrence of hot flashes.

STORAGE Keep in a convenient location.

TIP This blend helps with night sweats and insomnia, too. Address these issues by applying 2 drops of the blend to the sole of each foot while getting ready for bed.

Peppermint Neat Treatment

MAKES 1 TREATMENT

3 or 4 drops peppermint essential oil

Apply the peppermint essential oil to a cotton ball and swab your hairline when you feel a hot flash coming on, focusing on the area that extends from behind your ears to the back of your neck.

TIP If you are sensitive to peppermint essential oil, try spearmint instead.

IMPETIGO

Impetigo is a contagious infection of the skin's outer layers. First appearing as tiny red spots that enlarge and turn into blisters that break open, ooze pus, and develop a brownish-yellow crust, it usually occurs at the site of a minor injury or rash. Insect bites, poison ivy, eczema, and even little cuts and scrapes can allow the bacteria that causes impetigo to get under the skin; however, it also sometimes develops on healthy skin. Antibacterial essential oils such as lavender, myrrh, patchouli, and tea tree can bring relief while helping compromised skin heal.

Lavender Compress

MAKES ABOUT 1 OUNCE

1 ounce carrier oil

20 drops lavender essential oil

1. In a small bottle with a tight-fitting lid and an orifice reducer, combine the carrier oil with the lavender essential oil. Secure the lid and shake well to blend.
2. Using a cotton swab or a cotton ball, apply 2 drops of the blend to the affected area, using more or less as needed. Repeat three to four times daily.

STORAGE Keep in a cool, dark place.

TIP To treat those over 6 years, you can create a synergistic blend by adding 10 drops of tea tree essential oil.

Tea Tree Neat Treatment

6+

MAKES 1 TREATMENT

1 drop tea tree essential oil (per area)

Using a cotton swab, apply 1 drop of tea tree essential oil to each of the affected areas. Repeat twice daily.

TIP If you don't have tea tree essential oil, you can use eucalyptus instead.

INDIGESTION

Bloating, belching, and abdominal discomfort are a few of the most common symptoms of indigestion. Essential oils can bring relief while you take steps to identify and tackle the cause, which could be as simple as filling up on foods that disagree with you or as complex as gallbladder disease. Ginger essential oil is my go-to, and lemon, sweet orange, peppermint, and spearmint are some others to try.

Ginger Smelling Salts

MAKES ABOUT ½ OUNCE

1 tablespoon Epsom salt or Dead Sea salt

4 drops ginger essential oil

1. In a small jar with a tight-fitting lid, combine the salt with the ginger essential oil. Secure the lid and shake well to blend.

2. Inhale deeply from the jar as soon as discomfort begins. Add another 4 drops of ginger essential oil when the scent fades.

STORAGE Keep in a convenient location.

TIP If you don't have ginger essential oil, try this remedy with peppermint or spearmint.

Chamomile-Peppermint Balm

MAKES ABOUT 4 OUNCES

4 ounces carrier oil

30 drops peppermint essential oil

20 drops Roman chamomile essential oil

1. In a small bottle or jar with a tight-fitting lid, combine the carrier oil with the peppermint and Roman chamomile essential oils. Secure the lid and shake well to blend.
2. Apply ¼ teaspoon of the blend to your upper abdomen, focusing on the area located just below your sternum. Massage gently for two to three minutes, then lie on your left side for at least 10 minutes while relaxing. Repeat two to three times daily, or as needed.

STORAGE Keep in a convenient location if using frequently; otherwise, keep in a cool, dark place.

TIP If creating this blend for a child under 6 years, replace the peppermint essential oil with spearmint.

Sweet Orange–Lemon Massage Oil

MAKES ABOUT 1 OUNCE

1 ounce jojoba oil

20 drops sweet orange essential oil

20 drops lemon essential oil

1. In a small bottle or jar with a tight-fitting lid, combine the jojoba oil with the sweet orange and lemon essential oils. Secure the lid and shake well to blend.
2. Apply 3 or 4 drops of the blend to the sole of each foot, focusing on the arches and surrounding area. Repeat once or twice daily as needed.

STORAGE Keep in a cool, dark place.

TIP Try this blend for stress or tension. You can massage a bit into each temple or add 1 teaspoon to a warm bath.

INFLAMMATION

Inflammation is the body's response to threats. It can accompany viruses, fungal infections, and a variety of illnesses and injuries, manifesting as redness, irritation, swelling, heat, and pain. Although inflammation is part of the body's natural healing process, the pain that accompanies it can interfere with the enjoyment of everyday life. In some cases, such as autoimmune disease, inflammation creates widespread discomfort. Anti-inflammatory essential oils offer pain relief while helping the healing process along.

Thyme Diffusion

MAKES 1 TREATMENT

2 or 3 drops thyme essential oil

Following the manufacturer's instructions, add the thyme essential oil to your diffuser. Run the diffuser nearby. Repeat every two to three hours or as needed.

TIP Try thyme in vapor therapy, too. Use it in a humidifier or vaporizer, or add 4 drops of thyme essential oil to a hot bath.

Anti-inflammatory Clove Salve

MAKES ABOUT 4 OUNCES

4 ounces aloe vera gel

20 drops clove essential oil

1. In a small jar with a tight-fitting lid, combine the aloe gel with the clove essential oil. Stir well with a thin utensil.
2. Use a cotton ball to apply ¼ teaspoon of the salve to the affected area. Repeat two to three times daily.

STORAGE Keep in a cool, dark place.

TIP This salve can also bring quick relief to painful, itchy skin conditions. Clove causes a feeling of numbness, so don't apply it with your bare fingertips.

INGROWN HAIR

Ingrown hairs aren't just unsightly; they can also become red, swollen, and infected. Never squeeze or pick at an ingrown hair, as this can make matters worse. Exfoliate and reach for essential oil instead. Once the tip of the hair emerges, you can use a pair of pointed tweezers to tease it out into the open. Tea tree is my go-to for preventing infection, and lavender, lemongrass, frankincense, and Roman chamomile can work wonders, too.

Tea Tree Neat Treatment

MAKES 1 TREATMENT

1 drop tea tree essential oil

Exfoliate the affected area and then apply the tea tree essential oil directly to the ingrown hair. Repeat once daily until the ingrown hair emerges.

TIP If you don't have tea tree essential oil on hand, you can use lavender instead.

Lavender-Chamomile Sugar Scrub

MAKES ABOUT 8 OUNCES

¾ cup brown sugar

2 ounces extra-virgin olive oil

10 drops lavender essential oil

10 drops Roman chamomile essential oil

1. In a small jar with a tight-fitting lid, combine the brown sugar and olive oil with the lavender and Roman chamomile essential oils. Secure the lid and shake well to combine.
2. Spend 5 minutes in a warm shower or bath, then use your hands to apply 1 tablespoon of the sugar scrub to the affected areas. Use more or less of the scrub as needed.
3. Scrub using light, circular motions, rubbing until the sugar dissolves. Rinse thoroughly and pat yourself dry, then check the ingrown hairs to see if they have emerged. Repeat as needed to treat and prevent ingrown hairs.

STORAGE Keep in a cool, dark place.

TIP This sugar scrub is also fantastic for twice-weekly facial exfoliation. Use just ½ teaspoon on wet skin. After rinsing, your face will look fresh and feel smooth.

INGROWN TOENAIL

Ingrown toenails can make wearing shoes a painful proposition. Trimming nails properly can prevent this problem from occurring, but sometimes, despite your best efforts, you may find yourself with this condition. Without treatment, the redness and swelling will worsen. Certain essential oils can help ease discomfort and prevent infection after home treatment or while you're waiting to see the podiatrist. →

Lavender–Tea Tree Salve

MAKES ABOUT ⅓ OUNCE

2 teaspoons jojoba oil

20 drops lavender essential oil

20 drops tea tree essential oil

1. In a small bottle with a tight-fitting lid, combine the jojoba oil with the lavender and tea tree essential oils. Secure the lid and shake well to blend.
2. Use a cotton ball to apply 4 to 6 drops of the blend to the affected area. Repeat two to three times daily until the ingrown toenail is healed.

STORAGE Keep in a cool, dark place.

TIP This salve is a good one to use as a preventive for athlete's foot. Use 2 or 3 drops between the toes of each foot.

Frankincense Neat Treatment

MAKES 1 TREATMENT

1 drop frankincense essential oil

1. Wash the affected area with soap and water, and use a soft towel to dry it completely.
2. Gently pry the swollen skin away from the toenail. Holding it in place, apply the frankincense essential oil directly down into the affected area. Repeat twice daily.

TIP If you don't have frankincense on hand, try myrrh, lavender, or tea tree essential oil instead.

INSECT BITES

Mosquitos, midges, and other pests are often an unavoidable part of otherwise enjoyable outdoor experiences. The itchiness and the unsightly red bump that follows a bug bite come from a natural anticoagulant that the insect injects into your skin to prevent your blood from clotting while it feeds. Not only is this a bit icky, it also causes a mild allergic reaction. Essential oils with anti-inflammatory and analgesic properties bring relief while helping your skin recover faster.

Minty Lavender-Lemon Salve

MAKES ABOUT 2 OUNCES

2 ounces extra-virgin coconut oil, softened

20 drops spearmint essential oil

20 drops lavender essential oil

10 drops lemon essential oil

1. In a small jar with a tight-fitting lid, combine the coconut oil with the spearmint, lavender, and lemon essential oils. Stir well with a thin utensil.
2. Apply a pea-size amount to each insect bite. Use a little more or less if needed, and repeat the treatment two to three times daily.

STORAGE Keep in a cool, dark place.

TIP If you plan to spend time in the sun, omit the lemon essential oil. You can replace it with helichrysum, if you like.

Helichrysum Gel

MAKES ABOUT 4 OUNCES

4 ounces aloe vera gel

20 drops helichrysum essential oil

1. In a small jar with a tight-fitting lid, combine the aloe gel with the helichrysum essential oil. Stir well with a thin utensil.
2. Use a cotton swab or fingertip to apply a drop of gel to each insect bite. Repeat three to four times daily.

STORAGE Keep in a cool, dark place.

TIP This is a good all-purpose first-aid gel; use it on minor burns, cuts, and scrapes.

Niaouli Spray

MAKES ABOUT 8 OUNCES

8 ounces alcohol-free witch hazel

1 teaspoon niaouli essential oil

1. In a small bottle with a fine-mist spray top, combine the witch hazel with the niaouli essential oil, and secure the top. Shake well before each use.
2. Spritz the affected areas and allow them to dry before dressing. Repeat three to four times daily.

STORAGE Keep in a cool, dark place.

TIP If you don't have niaouli essential oil, you can use peppermint, spearmint, or eucalyptus instead.

INSOMNIA

Stress, anxiety, and excitement are a few factors that can lead to insomnia. Instead of risking unpleasant side effects by reaching for sleep aids, try essential oils with sedative properties. Lavender, chamomile, and ylang-ylang are a few of the best, encouraging deep relaxation so you can fall asleep effortlessly and wake up feeling refreshed. You can also help your body prepare for sleep by turning off electronics about an hour before bed.

Chamomile and Marjoram Aromatherapy

MAKES 1 TREATMENT

4 drops chamomile essential oil

4 drops marjoram essential oil

1. One hour before you prepare for bed, apply the chamomile and marjoram essential oils to a cotton ball. Keep the cotton ball nearby until you turn in for the night. (If you'd like, you can tuck it into your bra strap or put it in an upper pocket.)
2. When you lie down in bed, position the cotton ball a few feet from your face.

TIP Try this blend in a humidifier or vaporizer in your bedroom, or add the oils to a relaxing bedtime bath.

Energizing Lemongrass-Grapefruit Smelling Salts

MAKES ABOUT ½ OUNCE

1 tablespoon Epsom salt or Dead Sea salt

4 drops grapefruit essential oil

4 drops lemongrass essential oil

1. In a small jar with a tight-fitting lid, combine the salt with the grapefruit and lemongrass essential oils. Secure the lid and shake well to blend.
2. Inhale deeply from the jar anytime fatigue starts to set in. Add more essential oil when the scent fades.

STORAGE Keep in a convenient location.

TIP If you don't have grapefruit essential oil, try this remedy with lemon, sweet orange, or mandarin.

JOINT PAIN

Stiff, sore joints rarely require a doctor's visit. Assuming any serious causes have been ruled out, the prescribed remedy is usually an OTC pain reliever. But instead of reaching for those painkillers, which might lead to unwanted side effects, try giving analgesic essential oils a chance to relieve the discomfort. Pine, juniper, and peppermint are some of the best, penetrating deep to bring fast, fragrant relief.

Peppermint Neat Treatment

MAKES 1 TREATMENT

4 drops peppermint essential oil

Apply the peppermint essential oil directly to the painful joint. Repeat every three to four hours for up to three days.

TIP If treating a child under 6 years, use spearmint instead of peppermint, diluting 1:1 with a carrier oil.

Juniper-Pine Massage Oil

MAKES ABOUT 2 OUNCES

2 ounces jojoba oil

20 drops pine essential oil

20 drops juniper essential oil

1. In a small bottle with a tight-fitting lid, combine the jojoba oil with the pine and juniper essential oils. Secure the lid and shake well to blend.
2. Apply 3 or 4 drops of the blend to a cosmetic pad, and swab the affected joint, using more or less depending on the size of the joint. Repeat every two to three hours or as needed.

STORAGE Keep in a cool, dark place.

TIP This massage oil makes an excellent vapor treatment for treating colds and coughs. Put 1 teaspoon into a hot bath and breathe deeply while relaxing.

KERATOSIS PILARIS

Also known as chicken skin, keratosis pilaris typically affects the upper arms and legs. The condition occurs when a naturally occurring protein called keratin *clogs pores, and it can get worse in dry environments. The bumps don't normally cause discomfort, but they might lead to self-consciousness that prevents you from wearing the same sleeveless styles everyone else enjoys. Faithfully moisturizing, exfoliating, and using anti-inflammatory essential oils can work wonders so you can wear those shorts, sundresses, and tank tops you've been admiring from afar.*

Myrrh Moisturizing Cream

MAKES ABOUT 8 OUNCES

6 ounces shea butter

2 ounces jojoba oil

24 drops myrrh essential oil

1. In a small jar with a tight-fitting lid, combine the shea butter and jojoba oil with the myrrh essential oil. Stir well with a thin utensil.
2. Apply ¼ teaspoon of the cream to each affected area, massaging gently. Repeat once or twice daily.

STORAGE Keep in a cool, dark place.

TIP If you suffer from dry, scaly knees and elbows, this cream can help. Apply a pea-size amount to each area of dry skin and massage in.

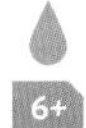

Geranium, Juniper, and Clary Sage Sugar Scrub

MAKES ABOUT 8 OUNCES

¾ cup brown sugar

2 ounces jojoba oil

10 drops geranium essential oil

10 drops juniper essential oil

10 drops clary sage essential oil

1. In a small jar with a tight-fitting lid, combine the brown sugar and jojoba oil with the geranium, juniper, and clary sage essential oils. Secure the lid and shake well to blend.
2. After showering for at least 5 minutes, step away from the showerhead and apply 1 teaspoon of the sugar scrub to each affected area. Using tight circular motions, massage each area until the sugar dissolves.
3. Rinse thoroughly. Pat dry, then moisturize before dressing. Repeat once daily.

STORAGE Keep in a cool, dark place.

TIP This blend makes a fantastic all-over body scrub that will leave your skin feeling soft and smooth.

LARYNGITIS

Whether it's caused by an infection or cheering for your favorite team until your throat feels raw, an inflamed larynx makes talking tough. Allergies, smoking, and coughing due to another illness are some other contributors. While laryngitis often clears up on its own, essential oils can make you more comfortable while your voice box heals. Staying warm, keeping hydrated, and avoiding irritants can keep the discomfort from getting worse.

Ginger Gargle

MAKES ABOUT 8 OUNCES

7 ounces distilled or purified water

1 ounce aloe vera gel

8 drops ginger essential oil

1. In a small bottle with a tight-fitting lid, combine the water and aloe gel with the ginger essential oil and secure the lid. Shake well before each use.
2. Gargle with 1 tablespoon of the solution two to three times daily, taking care not to swallow.

STORAGE Keep in a cool, dark place.

TIP Use ginger to treat children under 6 years by combining 12 drops of ginger essential oil with 1 ounce of carrier oil and then applying 3 or 4 drops of the blend to the throat area twice daily.

Thyme Vapor Treatment

MAKES 1 TREATMENT

2 cups steaming hot (not boiling) water

2 drops thyme essential oil

1. Pour the water into a shallow bowl and add the thyme essential oil.
2. Sitting comfortably in front of the bowl, drape a towel over your head and the bowl, creating a tent that concentrates the steam and vapors. Breathe deeply until the water cools and the vapors subside, emerging for cool air as needed. Repeat once or twice daily.

TIP As an alternative to the vapor tent for children under 12 years, diffuse the thyme essential oil a few feet away from the activity area or in the child's bedroom. A vaporizer or humidifier is another option.

Peppermint-Pine Massage Oil

MAKES ABOUT 2 OUNCES

2 ounces carrier oil

20 drops peppermint essential oil

10 drops pine essential oil

1. In a small bottle or jar with a tight-fitting lid, combine the carrier oil with the peppermint and pine essential oils. Secure the lid and shake well to blend. ➛

Peppermint-Pine Massage Oil continued

2. Apply ¼ teaspoon of the oil to the outside of your throat. Gently massage the soft tissue located on either side of your larynx with your fingertips. Use light strokes and massage for 5 to 10 minutes per session. Repeat the treatment once or twice daily until symptoms subside.

STORAGE Keep in a cool, dark place.

TIP If treating a child under 6 years, replace the peppermint and pine essential oils with your choice of 20 drops of spearmint or ginger.

LEG CRAMPS

While leg cramps aren't usually serious, they can cause debilitating pain. With sharp contractions and hard knots you can sometimes see, sudden leg cramps can leave you sore for hours after the episode ends. Analgesic and antispasmodic essential oils can increase circulation and provide quick pain relief. If your leg cramps happen frequently, be sure to see your doctor to rule out underlying medical causes.

Peppermint-Cypress Massage Oil

MAKES ABOUT 1 OUNCE

1 ounce jojoba oil

20 drops peppermint essential oil

10 drops cypress essential oil

1. In a small bottle or jar with a tight-fitting lid, combine the jojoba oil with the peppermint and cypress essential oils. Secure the lid and shake well to blend.
2. Starting at the ankle and working your way up your leg, use circular motions to massage 1 teaspoon of the blend into your leg. When you finish, massage your foot. Repeat as needed.

STORAGE Keep in a cool, dark place.

TIP You can use this remedy for cold and flu symptoms, too, by massaging ½ teaspoon of the blend into the chest and neck area two to three times daily.

Lavender-Marjoram Bath Salts

MAKES ABOUT 16 OUNCES

2 cups Epsom salt

10 drops lavender essential oil

20 drops marjoram essential oil

1. In a quart jar with a tight-fitting lid, combine the salt with the lavender and marjoram essential oils. Secure the lid and shake well to blend.
2. Draw a hot bath and dissolve ½ cup of the bath salts in it. Rest and relax for 30 minutes.

STORAGE Keep in a cool, dark place.

TIP This treatment is also excellent for lower back pain, postworkout discomfort, and menstrual cramps.

LICE

Discovering that your child has picked up head lice might seem like cause for panic, but essential oils make it easier to deal with an outbreak without resorting to harsh chemicals. Some essential oils, such as tea tree and geranium, are strong natural pesticides that also provide relief from itchy bites. Since children have sensitive scalps, it's important to dilute the essential oils well before application.

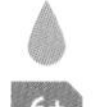

6+

Tea Tree Shampoo

MAKES ABOUT 4 OUNCES

4 ounces shampoo (any kind)
20 drops tea tree essential oil

1. In a small squeeze bottle, combine the shampoo with the tea tree essential oil. Secure the top and shake well to blend.
2. Apply 1 teaspoon of the shampoo to damp hair and scrub thoroughly. Leave the shampoo in place for 5 to 10 minutes, then rinse out.
3. Using a lice comb, carefully work your way through the hair in segments, removing any dead and dying lice. Repeat daily until all signs of lice are gone.

STORAGE Keep in a cool, dark place.

TIP This shampoo is also an excellent remedy for dandruff, scalp eczema, and scalp psoriasis. Use it once daily to bring relief.

Synergistic Delousing Blend

MAKES ABOUT 8 OUNCES

1 cup extra-virgin coconut oil, softened

6 drops tea tree essential oil

6 drops thyme essential oil

4 drops lavender essential oil

4 drops geranium essential oil

1. In a small jar with a tight-fitting lid, combine the coconut oil with the tea tree, thyme, lavender, and geranium essential oils. Stir well with a thin utensil.
2. Apply 1 tablespoon of the blend to the scalp, working it into the quarter- to half-inch of hair closest to the scalp, where lice lay their eggs. Leave the blend in place for 20 minutes, then rinse out.
3. Using a lice comb, carefully work your way through the hair in segments, removing any dead and dying lice. Repeat daily until all signs of lice are gone.

STORAGE Keep in a cool, dark place.

TIP This blend can also help treat fungal infections like athlete's foot and ringworm.

MENSTRUAL CRAMPS

The cramps you feel during your menstrual cycle are completely natural, but that doesn't mean they're easy to tolerate. Antispasmodic, analgesic, and emmenagogue essential oils ease discomfort without causing unpleasant side effects. You can use them on their own or with other remedies, including OTC analgesics, if necessary.

Peppermint-Cypress Pain Rub

MAKES ABOUT 4 OUNCES

4 ounces jojoba oil

20 drops peppermint essential oil

10 drops cypress essential oil

1. In a small bottle or jar with a tight-fitting lid, combine the jojoba oil with the peppermint and cypress essential oils. Secure the lid and shake well to blend.
2. Massage 1 teaspoon of the blend into your lower abdomen, then massage another teaspoon of the blend into your lower back. Repeat twice daily or as needed.

STORAGE Keep in a cool, dark place.

TIP This blend works wonders when applied to overworked feet. After bathing or showering, apply ½ teaspoon to each foot, massaging well.

Clary Sage Neat Treatment

MAKES 1 TREATMENT

3 or 4 drops clary sage essential oil

Apply the clary sage essential oil directly to your lower abdomen, focusing on the area where the pain is worst. Speed relief by covering the area with a towel and then applying a warm heating pad to the site.

TIP Add 3 or 4 drops of clary sage and an equal amount of chamomile essential oil to a hot bath to help with cramps and promote relaxation before you turn in for the night.

MIGRAINE

Unbearable pain, sensitivity to light, and debilitating nausea are some of the most common migraine symptoms. Cooling essential oils with analgesic properties can help bring rapid relief—especially if you use them at the first signs that a migraine is about to strike. Help speed relief by staying hydrated and relaxing in a dark, quiet place if possible. If stress or lack of sleep frequently leads to migraines, treat yourself to a bottle of ylang-ylang essential oil and diffuse a drop or two while relaxing in the evening. →

Minty Lavender-Lemon Vapor

MAKES 1 TREATMENT

6 drops peppermint essential oil

4 drops lavender essential oil

1. Apply the peppermint and lavender essential oils to a washcloth. Place the cloth in the shower at the end opposite the showerhead.
2. In the shower, begin with warm water and gradually increase the heat while inhaling deeply. Gradually reduce the temperature until the water is cold, then gradually bring it back to hot. Repeat the cycle two or three times, ending with a burst of cold.

TIP If the idea of cold water splashing down on you doesn't sound appealing or if you find that it doesn't improve your circulation, you can use just the combination of warm and hot water.

Peppermint-Marjoram Migraine Massage Oil

MAKES ABOUT ½ OUNCE

2 teaspoons carrier oil

30 drops peppermint essential oil

20 drops marjoram essential oil

1. In a small bottle with a tight-fitting lid and an orifice reducer, combine the carrier oil with the peppermint and marjoram essential oils. Secure the lid and shake well to blend.

2. Apply 1 drop of the blend to each of your temples and gently massage it in. Then apply 3 drops to the back of your neck, massaging it into your hairline. Repeat two to three times daily.

STORAGE Keep in a convenient location.

TIP You can also apply this blend to the bottoms of your feet before lying down to relax. Focus on the pads of your toes and the underside of each of your big toes. These reflexology points correspond with your frontal sinuses and your brain.

Peppermint-Rosemary Diffusion

MAKES 1 TREATMENT

3 drops rosemary essential oil

2 drops peppermint essential oil

Following the manufacturer's instructions, add the rosemary and peppermint essential oils to your diffuser. Run the diffuser nearby. Repeat every two to three hours or as needed.

TIP This blend is excellent for vapor therapy, too. Use it in a humidifier or vaporizer, or drip the rosemary and peppermint essential oils onto a washcloth, bring it into the shower, and place it opposite the showerhead.

MORNING SICKNESS

Morning sickness symptoms can take some of the joy out of your pregnancy, particularly during the first trimester, when they're at their worst. Lemongrass and spearmint essential oils are among the few that are safe to use during pregnancy. With their fresh, uplifting fragrances and digestive properties, they can help put a stop to vomiting.

Spearmint Smelling Salts

MAKES ABOUT ½ OUNCE

1 tablespoon coarse salt

10 drops spearmint essential oil

1. In a small bottle with a tight-fitting lid, combine the salt with the spearmint essential oil. Secure the lid and shake well to blend.
2. As soon as you feel stomach acid rising, inhale deeply from the bottle for two to three minutes. Use as often as needed. Add more spearmint essential oil when the scent fades.

STORAGE Keep in a convenient location.

TIP This treatment is also ideal for young children suffering from motion sickness, nausea, or vomiting.

Lemongrass-Spearmint Diffusion

MAKES 1 TREATMENT

5 drops spearmint essential oil

2 drops lemongrass essential oil

Following the manufacturer's instructions, add the spearmint and lemongrass essential oils to your diffuser. Run the diffuser at bedtime. Repeat nightly. Within three nights, the urge to vomit in the morning should subside.

TIP You can also use this blend for vapor therapy. Use it in a humidifier or vaporizer, or drip the spearmint and lemongrass essential oils onto a washcloth, bring it into the shower, and place it opposite the showerhead.

MOTION SICKNESS

Nausea and vomiting can take all the fun out of road trips, scenic ocean cruises, and air travel. Instead of relying on OTC remedies that can put you to sleep, try these simple treatments. Thanks to its powerful antinausea action, ginger is my favorite essential oil for dealing with motion sickness, but others may respond better to Roman chamomile, peppermint, or spearmint. With just a bit of experimentation, you'll quickly find the remedy that suits you best. →

Ginger Smelling Salts

MAKES ABOUT ½ OUNCE

1 tablespoon coarse salt

10 drops ginger essential oil

1. In a small bottle with a tight-fitting lid, combine the salt with the ginger essential oil. Secure the lid and shake well to blend.
2. Inhale deeply from the bottle for two to three minutes. Use as often as needed. Add more ginger essential oil when the scent fades.

STORAGE Keep in a convenient location.

TIP In a pinch, you can place a drop or two of ginger essential oil on a tissue or handkerchief and inhale until the nausea fades.

Spearmint Neat Treatment

MAKES 1 TREATMENT

2 drops spearmint essential oil

Apply 1 drop of spearmint essential oil behind each ear 15 to 30 minutes before departure. Repeat every three to four hours if necessary.

TIP Treat cranky, nauseous children by dabbing 3 drops each of spearmint and Roman chamomile essential oils onto a favorite stuffed toy. Encourage them to hold the toy while traveling, and tuck it in close to them if they tire of holding it.

MUSCLE SORENESS

Physical exertion often leads to muscle pain and tenderness. Even though a good workout may be worth it, there's no reason to suffer. Essential oils bring fast relief by penetrating the skin and blocking pain. Peppermint and spearmint are popular solutions, but warming, spicy oils such as ginger and clove work well, too, especially when used in topical remedies and baths.

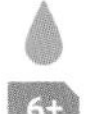

Clary Sage–Juniper Spray

MAKES ABOUT 4 OUNCES

2 ounces alcohol-free witch hazel

1 ounce aloe vera gel

1 ounce jojoba oil

20 drops clary sage essential oil

10 drops juniper essential oil

1. In a small bottle with a fine-mist spray top, combine the witch hazel, aloe gel, and jojoba oil with the clary sage and juniper essential oils. Secure the top and shake well before each use.
2. Spritz areas of muscle soreness once or twice and then massage until the blend is absorbed.

STORAGE Keep in a cool, dark place.

TIP You can also use this blend to soothe irritated or inflamed skin by applying a few drops to the affected area with a cotton ball, repeating twice daily as needed.

Ginger-Clove Balm

MAKES ABOUT 1 OUNCE

1 ounce extra-virgin coconut oil, softened

20 drops ginger essential oil

20 drops clove essential oil

1. In a small jar with a tight-fitting lid, combine the coconut oil with the ginger and clove essential oils. Stir well with a thin utensil.
2. Apply ¼ teaspoon of the blend to areas of muscle soreness. Repeat every two to three hours or as needed.

STORAGE Keep in a cool, dark place.

TIP If you don't have ginger or clove, make a cooling pain relief balm by mixing 40 drops of peppermint essential oil with the coconut oil instead.

Peppermint Neat Treatment

MAKES 1 TREATMENT

4 drops peppermint essential oil

Apply the peppermint essential oil directly to the painful area, using more or less as needed. Repeat two to three times daily until soreness subsides.

TIP If you don't have peppermint essential oil, try this treatment with lavender instead. Although it doesn't relieve pain as quickly, it does offer some relief.

MUSCLE SPASMS

Painful and irritating, muscle spasms happen when tissue is overworked, overstretched, or inflamed; sometimes the problem is caused by low electrolytes, dehydration, or a mineral deficiency. Antispasmodic, analgesic, and anti-inflammatory essential oils help by penetrating the skin and entering the tissue and bloodstream beneath, where they provide a pleasant warming sensation. Marjoram is my go-to for muscle spasms, but there are others that work well, too. Give lavender, Roman chamomile, rosemary, or clary sage a try.

Lavender–Clary Sage Compress

MAKES 1 TREATMENT

4 drops carrier oil

4 drops lavender essential oil

4 drops clary sage essential oil

1. In a small bowl, combine the carrier oil with the lavender and clary sage essential oils. Saturate a cotton pad with the blend, apply it to the affected area, and cover with a towel.
2. Place a warm heating pad over the towel and leave it in place for 10 to 15 minutes. Repeat every two to three hours or as needed.

TIP If you don't have time for a compress, you can simply apply the blend as a muscle rub.

Marjoram Neat Treatment

MAKES 1 TREATMENT

2 or 3 drops marjoram essential oil

Apply the marjoram essential oil directly to the affected area. Repeat as often as needed.

TIP For whole-body relaxation, add ½ cup of Epsom salt and 6 drops of marjoram essential oil to a tub of hot water and soak for 15 minutes.

MUSCLE STIFFNESS

Overuse, repetitive motion, and even long hours spent sitting at your desk can lead to muscle stiffness. Not only is this condition uncomfortable, it makes everyday activities difficult. Instead of reaching for pain meds, try essential oils with analgesic or anti-inflammatory properties. Peppermint, lavender, and thyme are some of my favorites; when there's time, adding them to a bath or covering them with a hot compress can speed relief.

Peppermint-Thyme Salve

MAKES ABOUT 4 OUNCES

4 ounces carrier oil

15 drops peppermint essential oil

15 drops thyme essential oil

1. In a small bottle or jar with a tight-fitting lid, combine the carrier oil with the peppermint and thyme essential oils. Secure the lid and shake well to combine.
2. Apply ¼ teaspoon of the salve to the affected area, massaging well. Repeat every two to three hours or as needed.

STORAGE Keep in a cool, dark place.

TIP For children under 6 years, replace the peppermint essential oil with spearmint.

Lavender-Cypress Bath Salts

MAKES ABOUT 16 OUNCES

2 cups Epsom salt

2 tablespoons carrier oil

20 drops lavender essential oil

10 drops cypress essential oil

1. In a quart jar with a tight-fitting lid, combine the salt and carrier oil with the lavender and cypress essential oils. Secure the lid and shake well to combine.
2. Draw a hot bath and add ½ cup of the bath salts. Spend 15 to 30 minutes relaxing.

STORAGE Keep in a cool, dark place.

TIP You can try this bath blend for body aches associated with cold and flu, too.

NAIL FUNGUS

Nail fungus isn't just an unsightly cosmetic issue; it's a highly contagious condition that can be difficult to treat. OTC remedies can cause undesirable side effects that you won't experience with antifungal essential oils. Treatment will go faster if you address fungus as soon as you notice discoloration, but with a consistent effort, you can get even serious fungal infections to clear up. Keeping your nails clean and dry can also help speed the healing process.

Antifungal Nail Soak

MAKES 1 TREATMENT

1 gallon lukewarm water

½ cup hydrogen peroxide

1 tablespoon carrier oil

10 drops tea tree essential oil

2 drops clove essential oil

1. Pour the water into a basin and add the peroxide, carrier oil, and tea tree and clove essential oils. Soak the affected hands or feet for 10 to 15 minutes.
2. Pat dry with a towel. Repeat daily until the fungus is gone.

TIP Make an antifungal spray for your home by omitting the carrier oil and peroxide. Blend the tea tree and clove essential oils with 16 ounces of water in a medium bottle with a fine-mist spray top and secure the lid. Shake well before each use. Spritz damp areas such as the kitchen and bathroom.

Tea Tree Neat Treatment

MAKES 1 TREATMENT

1 drop tea tree essential oil (per nail)

Apply the tea tree essential oil directly to each affected nail.

TIP Tea tree essential oil has an intense drying effect. If you have brittle nails, blend the tea tree 1:1 with a carrier oil. Repeat two to three times daily, continuing once-daily treatments after the fungus disappears.

NAUSEA

Digestive problems, morning sickness, stress, and cancer treatments are some of the most common causes of nausea. Essential oils can help you safely treat the problem without any unpleasant side effects. Often just inhaling the vapors from ginger or peppermint essential oil is enough to stop you running for the nearest restroom. If you are pregnant, try inhaling spearmint or orange instead, or try the pregnancy-safe morning sickness remedies beginning on page 166. Try topical applications for long-lasting relief or to prepare yourself for a situation that's likely to leave you feeling sick. →

Peppermint Neat Treatment

6+

MAKES 1 TREATMENT

4 to 6 drops peppermint essential oil

1. Wash and dry your feet, then apply 2 or 3 drops of peppermint essential oil onto each foot.
2. Elevate your feet and relax while the oil absorbs.

TIP When taking off your shoes is inconvenient, apply 1 drop of peppermint essential oil to the inside of each wrist. Replace the peppermint with spearmint essential oil for pregnant women and children under 6 years.

Ginger Massage Oil

MAKES 1 TREATMENT

1 teaspoon carrier oil

6 drops ginger essential oil

1. In a small bowl, combine the carrier oil with the ginger essential oil. Stir well with a thin utensil.
2. Saturate a cotton ball with the oil mixture, apply the entire amount to your upper abdomen, and massage with light pressure.

TIP If you don't have ginger, use peppermint or spearmint essential oil instead.

NIGHT TERRORS

Night terrors leave children in a twilight zone between sleep and wakefulness, often crying, moaning, or even screaming and thrashing. Sedative essential oils can reduce the severity of the problem, and in some cases, they can prevent night terrors and the sleepwalking that sometimes accompanies them. You can increase the effectiveness of these remedies by ensuring that your child isn't consuming caffeine or eating too much sugar, and is sticking to a regular sleep schedule. Turning off electronics an hour before bed will help, too.

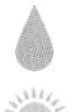

Sweet Orange–Thyme Bedtime Balm

MAKES ABOUT 4 OUNCES

4 ounces unscented body lotion

12 drops sweet orange essential oil

12 drops thyme essential oil

1. In a small jar with a tight-fitting lid, combine the body lotion with the sweet orange and thyme essential oils. Stir well with a thin utensil.
2. Apply 1 teaspoon of the balm to the child's hands and arms at bedtime.

STORAGE Keep in a cool, dark place.

TIP If your child usually spends daylight hours playing in the sun, replace the sweet orange with lavender essential oil.

Frankincense Diffusion

MAKES 1 TREATMENT

3 drops frankincense essential oil

Following the manufacturer's instructions, add the frankincense essential oil to your diffuser. Run the diffuser in your child's bedroom at night. Repeat nightly.

TIP If you don't have frankincense essential oil, use lavender instead.

NOSEBLEED

Nosebleeds result from broken blood vessels in the nose and can happen out of the blue—especially when you're exposed to hot, dry air. Essential oils can help by shrinking swollen tissue and promoting faster healing. While just one of these remedies will help a nosebleed, it's best to use both of them. Apply the compress first, and follow up with the gel.

Cypress Compress for Nosebleed

MAKES 1 TREATMENT

1 tablespoon cold water

4 drops cypress essential oil

1. Moisten a small cloth with the water and then add the cypress essential oil. Lay the cloth across your nose and cover it with an ice pack. Use your nondominant hand to keep the compress in place.

2. Sit comfortably, tipping your head slightly forward while pinching the soft part of your nose with the thumb and forefinger of your dominant hand. Keep pinching and holding the compress in place for 10 to 15 minutes.

TIP This treatment can be challenging for children. You can help them by having them pinch their nose while you hold the compress in place.

Comforting Helichrysum Gel

MAKES 1 TREATMENT

1 drop aloe vera gel

1 drop helichrysum essential oil

1. After the bleeding has stopped, in a small dish, combine the aloe gel and helichrysum essential oil. Use a cotton swab to blend, then scoop up as much gel as you can get on the tip of the swab.
2. Gently apply the gel to the inside of the affected nostril, focusing on the source of the blood flow. If possible, rest quietly for the next two to three hours.

TIP If you don't have helichrysum essential oil, you can use lavender in its place.

OILY SKIN

While oily skin is completely natural, the shininess and sticky, heavy feeling that accompany it can be overwhelming. Astringent essential oils cut through the oil, improving skin's appearance and helping you feel more comfortable. At the same time, they help prevent and treat the acne that tends to plague those with oily skin.

Lemon–Tea Tree Mask

MAKES 1 TREATMENT

1 teaspoon honey

3 drops lemon essential oil

1 drop tea tree essential oil

1. In the palm of your hand, combine the honey with the lemon and tea tree essential oils. Apply the blend to your freshly washed, dry face, and leave it in place for at least 10 minutes.
2. Rinse your face with warm water until the mask is completely washed away, and pat dry. Repeat two to three times weekly.

TIP If you plan to spend time in the sun, replace the lemon with lavender essential oil.

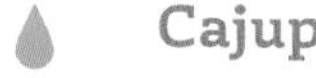

Cajuput Toner

MAKES ABOUT 8 OUNCES

8 ounces alcohol-free witch hazel

1 teaspoon cajuput essential oil

1. In a small bottle with a tight-fitting lid, combine the witch hazel with the cajuput essential oil. Secure the lid and shake well to blend.
2. With a cotton pad, apply ¼ teaspoon of the toner to your freshly washed face. Repeat once or twice daily.

STORAGE Keep in a cool, dark place.

TIP If you don't have cajuput, try an equal amount of tea tree or lavender essential oil instead.

Bergamot–Ylang-Ylang Night Cream

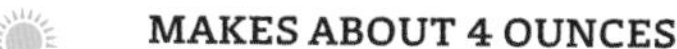

MAKES ABOUT 4 OUNCES

4 ounces oil-free facial moisturizer

12 drops ylang-ylang essential oil

6 drops bergamot essential oil

1. In a small jar with a tight-fitting lid, combine the moisturizer with the ylang-ylang and bergamot essential oils. Stir well with a thin utensil.
2. Apply ¼ teaspoon of the cream to your freshly washed face. Repeat each evening before bed.

STORAGE Keep in a cool, dark place.

TIP Make a daytime moisturizer for oily skin by replacing the ylang-ylang and bergamot essential oils with 16 drops of niaouli.

PNEUMONIA

You might be surprised to learn that there are more than 30 different types of pneumonia. Essential oils are suitable for mild types such as walking pneumonia, helping support the immune system so the lungs can heal. If your doctor agrees, consider using these treatments alongside conventional therapies. While essential oils won't cure your pneumonia, they can help you breathe a little easier.

Frankincense Diffusion

MAKES 1 TREATMENT

4 drops frankincense essential oil

Following the manufacturer's instructions, add the frankincense essential oil to your diffuser. Run the diffuser nearby. Repeat every two to three hours or as needed.

TIP Frankincense vapor therapy is a good bedtime alternative to diffusion; add 4 to 6 drops of frankincense essential oil to a humidifier or vaporizer.

Peppermint-Frankincense Chest Rub

MAKES ABOUT 4 OUNCES

4 ounces extra-virgin coconut oil, softened

20 drops frankincense essential oil

10 drops peppermint essential oil

1. In a small jar with a tight-fitting lid, combine the coconut oil with the frankincense and peppermint essential oils. Stir well with a thin utensil.
2. Apply ½ teaspoon of the rub to your chest and neck. Repeat every three to four hours or as needed.

STORAGE Keep in a cool, dark place.

TIP Treat children under 6 years by replacing the peppermint essential oil with spearmint.

POISON IVY OR POISON OAK

A run-in with poison ivy, poison oak, or poison sumac leaves you with a burning rash that can spread to other parts of your body if you aren't careful. The culprit is a compound called urushiol, *a colorless, odorless oil that protects the plants from predation. Peppermint essential oil is my go-to for poison ivy exposure. You can also use tea tree, lavender, or a combination of all three. They work by cutting through the urushiol, easing pain and itching, and helping the rash heal faster.*

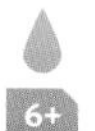

Peppermint–Tea Tree Spray for Poison Ivy

6+

MAKES ABOUT 4 OUNCES

4 ounces alcohol-free witch hazel

20 drops peppermint essential oil

20 drops tea tree essential oil →

Peppermint–Tea Tree Spray for Poison Ivy continued

1. In a small bottle with a fine-mist spray top, combine the witch hazel with the peppermint and tea tree essential oils and secure the top. Shake well before each use.
2. Spritz each affected area once every four to six hours or as needed.

STORAGE Keep in a cool, dark place.

TIP Treat children under 6 years by replacing the peppermint essential oil with spearmint.

Soothing Lavender–Tea Tree Oatmeal Bath

MAKES 1 TREATMENT

1 single-use packet unscented oatmeal bath powder

½ cup baking soda

10 drops lavender essential oil

10 drops tea tree essential oil

1. Draw a warm bath and add the oatmeal powder. Stir it in with your hand, breaking up any lumps, then add the baking soda.
2. Add the lavender and tea tree essential oils, and soak until the water cools. Pat yourself completely dry and dress comfortably.

TIP This bath works well for rashes, chicken pox, and hives, too.

POSTPARTUM DEPRESSION

Low hormone levels, anemia, and thyroiditis are some factors that can contribute to postpartum depression. Essential oils can help you cope with symptoms such as fatigue and feelings of sadness, but they don't address the underlying imbalances. While mild postpartum depression often resolves itself within 10 to 12 days of childbirth, serious cases require medical intervention. Seek professional help if your symptoms are severe or last longer than two weeks.

Lavender, Grapefruit, and Ylang-Ylang Diffusion

MAKES 1 TREATMENT

3 drops grapefruit essential oil

1 drop lavender essential oil

1 drop ylang-ylang essential oil

Following the manufacturer's instructions, add the grapefruit, lavender, and ylang-ylang essential oils to your diffuser. Run the diffuser nearby. Repeat every two to three hours or as needed.

TIP Try this balancing blend in a humidifier or vaporizer, or drip the grapefruit, lavender, and ylang-ylang essential oils onto a washcloth and enjoy it in the shower. Simply place the cloth opposite the showerhead.

Bergamot Balm

MAKES ABOUT ½ OUNCE

1 tablespoon carrier oil

20 drops bergamot essential oil

1. In a small bottle with a tight-fitting lid and an orifice reducer, combine the carrier oil with the bergamot essential oil. Secure the lid and shake well to blend.
2. Massage 1 drop of balm into each of your temples. Repeat every three to four hours or as needed.

STORAGE Keep in a convenient location.

TIP Try this fragrant balm whenever you feel stressed, anxious, or drained. It can help with cold and flu symptoms, too.

PREMENSTRUAL SYNDROME (PMS)

You can blame hormones for PMS. When progesterone levels drop to prepare the body for menstruation, it sets off a chain reaction that affects salt and sugar levels, which in turn leads to those familiar, but annoying, symptoms: headaches, irritability, water retention, and more. Essential oils can't put an end to PMS forever, but they do a marvelous job of helping eliminate or reduce the symptoms. Bergamot, clary sage, geranium, and Roman chamomile are some of the best to try.

Bergamot Vapor

MAKES 1 TREATMENT

2 cups steaming hot (not boiling) water

3 drops bergamot essential oil

1. Pour the water into a shallow bowl and add the bergamot essential oil.
2. Sitting comfortably in front of the bowl, drape a towel over your head and the bowl, creating a tent that concentrates the steam and vapors. Breathe deeply until the water cools and the vapors subside, emerging for cool air as needed. Repeat once or twice daily.

TIP Use this treatment to improve your mood anytime, but especially when you're feeling irritated or frustrated.

Lavender–Clary Sage Balm

MAKES ABOUT ½ OUNCE

1 tablespoon carrier oil

20 drops lavender essential oil

20 drops clary sage essential oil

1. In a small bottle with a tight-fitting lid and an orifice reducer, combine the carrier oil with the lavender and clary sage essential oils. Secure the lid and shake well to blend.
2. Massage 1 drop of the blend into each of your temples. Repeat every two to three hours or as needed. →

Lavender–Clary Sage Balm continued

STORAGE: Keep in a cool, dark place.

TIP If you're feeling really overwhelmed and have time, eliminate stress and discomfort by adding 4 to 6 drops of this blend to a hot bath. Spend at least 10 minutes relaxing.

Triple Aromatherapy Massage Oil

MAKES ABOUT 4 OUNCES

4 ounces carrier oil

20 drops clary sage essential oil

10 drops geranium essential oil

10 drops juniper essential oil

1. In a small bottle or jar with a tight-fitting lid, combine the carrier oil with the clary sage, geranium, and juniper essential oils. Secure the lid and shake well to blend.
2. Apply ½ teaspoon of the blend to your lower abdomen and massage until completely absorbed.

STORAGE Keep in a cool, dark place.

TIP A teaspoon of this blend in a hot bath will help you relax and improve your mood anytime.

PSORIASIS

Stress, sunburn, and other factors can bring on a psoriasis flare-up, complete with red, scaly patches that typically show up on the knees, elbows, arms, legs, back, and scalp. The itching and burning can be intense, and while essential oils don't cure psoriasis, they can bring reliable relief. Cedarwood, cajuput, juniper, and geranium are among the best to try. If you're experiencing a breakout that covers a small area, a cold compress can ease symptoms quickly.

Cedarwood-Juniper Massage Oil

MAKES ABOUT 4 OUNCES

4 ounces extra-virgin coconut oil, softened

20 drops cedarwood essential oil

15 drops juniper essential oil

1. In a small jar with a tight-fitting lid, combine the coconut oil with the cedarwood and juniper essential oils. Stir well with a thin utensil.
2. Apply ¼ teaspoon of the blend to each affected area, using a little more or less to ensure that all psoriasis patches are covered. Repeat every three to four hours or as needed.

STORAGE Keep in a cool, dark place.

TIP This blend also makes a great massage oil for tired joints and muscles.

Cold Cajuput Compress

MAKES 1 TREATMENT

¼ teaspoon carrier oil

3 drops cajuput essential oil

1. In the palm of your hand, combine the carrier oil with the cajuput essential oil. Rub your hands together briefly and apply directly to the affected area.
2. Cover the affected area with a soft cloth and then apply an ice pack. Leave the compress in place for 10 minutes. Repeat twice daily or as needed.

TIP Treat a sore throat by applying the blend to the chest and throat area and skipping the ice pack.

RAZOR BUMPS

Shaving is supposed to result in smooth-feeling skin, so it's understandably annoying when razor bumps appear. Yes, they are unsightly, but more important, they can easily become inflamed and infected. Essential oils bring quick relief from the itching and stinging, and thanks to their antibacterial activity, they can help prevent infection. Lavender is my go-to for this problem, either neat or blended into a soothing, moisturizing balm.

Lavender Balm

MAKES ABOUT 4 OUNCES

4 ounces aloe vera gel

16 drops lavender essential oil

1. In a small jar with a tight-fitting lid, combine the aloe gel with the lavender essential oil. Stir well with a thin utensil.
2. Apply ¼ teaspoon of the gel to each affected area. Repeat twice daily.

STORAGE Keep in a cool, dark place.

TIP This treatment works well for acne, too. Applying it once or twice daily clears up breakouts quickly.

Myrrh Toner

MAKES ABOUT 4 OUNCES

4 ounces alcohol-free witch hazel

20 drops myrrh essential oil

1. In a small bottle or jar with a tight-fitting lid, combine the witch hazel with the myrrh essential oil and secure the lid. Shake well before each use.
2. Use a cotton ball or cotton pad to apply 3 or 4 drops to each affected area.

STORAGE Keep in a cool, dark place.

TIP This toner can also be used to treat athlete's foot. Apply a few drops to the infected areas three to four times daily to stop itching and promote healing.

RESTLESS LEGS SYNDROME

This condition is characterized by involuntary twitching that starts shortly after getting into bed, preventing you from falling asleep. Sedative essential oils bring quick relief, and when you combine them with daily exercise, you may be able to stop your symptoms altogether. Serious cases of restless legs syndrome can be indicative of an underlying problem such as diabetes or anemia. See your doctor to rule out underlying causes if your symptoms are frequent or severe.

Chamomile-Lavender Lotion

MAKES ABOUT 4 OUNCES

4 ounces unscented body lotion

20 drops chamomile essential oil

20 drops lavender essential oil

1. In a small jar with a tight-fitting lid, combine the body lotion with the chamomile and lavender essential oils. Stir well with a thin utensil.
2. Just before you get into bed, massage 1 teaspoon of the lotion into each leg, using a little more if needed. Repeat nightly.

STORAGE Keep in a cool, dark place.

TIP This relaxing lotion can help with insomnia, too.

Calming Aromatherapy Bath

MAKES ABOUT 16 OUNCES

2 cups Epsom salt

20 drops frankincense essential oil

15 drops marjoram essential oil

15 drops clary sage essential oil

8 drops ylang-ylang essential oil

1. In a quart jar with a tight-fitting lid, combine the salt with the frankincense, marjoram, clary sage, and ylang-ylang essential oils. Secure the lid and shake well to blend.
2. Draw a warm bath and dissolve ½ cup of the bath salts in the water. Spend at least 15 minutes soaking. Repeat nightly or as needed.

STORAGE Keep in a cool, dark place.

TIP Use these bath salts anytime you're feeling stressed. They're also fantastic for easing PMS symptoms.

RINGWORM

Ringworm's icky name gives the impression that its raised, ring-shaped patches are caused by a creepy parasite; instead, fungus is to blame. Antifungal essential oils help stop ringworm fast, easing the intense itching and redness while killing the fungus. Tea tree oil works very quickly, but it can dry sensitive skin. Use the moisturizing Lavender-Thyme Salve if you find that tea tree is a little too strong. →

Tea Tree Neat Treatment

MAKES 1 TREATMENT

1 drop tea tree essential oil (per area)

Using a cotton swab, apply the tea tree essential oil to the affected area. Use a new swab for each area of infection. Repeat two to three times daily.

TIP If you feel an itchy area developing but don't see any redness, apply a dab of tea tree anyway. This can prevent a new spot from forming.

Lavender-Thyme Salve

MAKES ABOUT 1 OUNCE

1 ounce extra-virgin coconut oil, softened

30 drops lavender essential oil

30 drops thyme essential oil

20 drops tea tree essential oil

1. In a small jar with a tight-fitting lid, combine the coconut oil with the lavender, thyme, and tea tree essential oils. Stir well with a thin utensil.
2. Using a cotton swab, apply a pea-size amount of the salve to each affected area. Use a new swab for each area you treat. Repeat two or three times daily.

STORAGE Keep in a cool, dark place.

TIP This salve has strong anti-inflammatory properties; use it to help bruises heal faster, too.

Triple Aromatherapy Spray

MAKES ABOUT 4 OUNCES

4 ounces alcohol-free witch hazel

20 drops lavender essential oil

10 drops lemongrass essential oil

10 drops thyme essential oil

1. In a small bottle with a fine-mist spray top, combine the witch hazel with the lavender, lemongrass, and thyme essential oils. Secure the top and shake well to blend.
2. Spritz once on each affected area, spritzing a little more if needed. Repeat two to three times daily.

STORAGE Keep in a cool, dark place.

TIP If the affected area is small, you may find it more convenient to apply this blend with a cotton swab rather than spraying it on.

SHINGLES

Shingles occur when the virus that causes chicken pox reactivates, resulting in painful red patches and blisters. Cases range from mild to severe, and the pain can be quite intense. Strong, analgesic essential oils help with the pain and itching, but they can't cure the disease. If your symptoms get worse instead of better, see your doctor. Severe shingles outbreaks often require medical intervention. ➛

Geranium Neat Treatment

MAKES 1 TREATMENT

1 or 2 drops geranium essential oil (per area)

Using a cotton swab or cotton pad, apply geranium essential oil to each affected area. Repeat twice daily.

TIP You can also use this treatment to help deep, painful bruises heal faster.

Clove Spray

MAKES ABOUT 4 OUNCES

3 ounces alcohol-free witch hazel

1 ounce aloe vera gel

20 drops clove essential oil

1. In a small bottle with a fine-mist spray top, combine the witch hazel and aloe gel with the clove essential oil and secure the top. Shake well before each use.
2. Spray a small amount of the solution onto each of the affected areas. Repeat two to three times daily.

STORAGE Keep in a cool, dark place.

TIP Spritz a little of this spray on insect bites, too, to bring quick relief.

SINUSITIS

A persistent stuffy nose, painful sinus pressure, and headaches certainly make daily tasks more difficult. If you're dealing with this condition, antiseptic and antibacterial essential oils can help by easing symptoms without causing unwanted side effects. My favorite sinus helpers are rosemary and thyme, especially as a blend. Eucalyptus, tea tree, and niaouli are some other good ones to try.

Rosemary-Thyme Vapor

MAKES 1 TREATMENT

2 cups steaming hot (not boiling) water

2 drops rosemary essential oil

1 drop thyme essential oil

1. Pour the water into a shallow bowl and add the rosemary and thyme essential oils.
2. Sitting comfortably in front of the bowl (with a box of tissues nearby), drape a towel over your head and the bowl, creating a tent that concentrates the steam and vapors. Breathe deeply until the water cools and the vapors subside, emerging to blow your nose as needed. Repeat once daily.

TIP If you'd like to multitask or watch TV during the treatment, you can place the rosemary and thyme essential oils in a vaporizer or humidifier instead.

Niaouli Diffusion

MAKES 1 TREATMENT

3 drops niaouli essential oil

Following the manufacturer's instructions, add the niaouli essential oil to your diffuser. Run the diffuser in your bedroom. Repeat nightly.

TIP If you don't have a diffuser, you can create an aromatic niaouli room spray by combining 4 ounces of distilled or purified water with 16 drops of niaouli essential oil in a small bottle with a fine-mist spray top. Shake well before each use.

Ginger-Myrrh Sinus Massage Oil

MAKES ABOUT 1 OUNCE

1 ounce carrier oil

10 drops myrrh essential oil

6 drops ginger essential oil

1. In a small bottle with a tight-fitting lid and an orifice reducer, combine the carrier oil with the myrrh and ginger essential oils. Secure the lid and shake well to blend.
2. Apply 4 drops of the oil to your fingertips. Using small circular motions, gently massage your sinus area for one to two minutes. Apply a little more if needed. Repeat two to three times daily.

STORAGE Keep in a cool, dark place.

TIP If you have oily skin, you can replace the carrier oil with the same amount of aloe vera gel.

SORE THROAT

Often among the first signs that the flu or a cold is imminent, a sore throat can begin as a little tickle that quickly gives way to burning pain. While essential oils don't usually eliminate throat pain permanently, they offer rapid, reliable relief. If you suspect that you have something more serious than a cold or a minor case of the flu, consider seeing your doctor for something stronger. Since sore throat also accompanies strep, it's possible you may need antibiotics.

Clove Gargle for Sore Throat

MAKES ABOUT 8 OUNCES

7 ounces distilled or purified water

1 ounce unflavored vodka

16 drops clove essential oil

1. In a small bottle or jar with a tight-fitting lid, combine the water and vodka with the clove essential oil, and secure the lid. Shake well before each use.
2. Gargle with 1 tablespoon of the solution twice daily, taking care not to swallow.

STORAGE Keep in a cool, dark place.

TIP To make an alcohol-free version, replace the vodka with one more ounce of distilled or purified water. This substitution is also suitable for kids 6 years and older, so long as parents supervise and are confident the child can gargle safely without swallowing.

Cajuput Aromatherapy Treatment

6+

MAKES 1 TREATMENT

2 drops cajuput essential oil

1. Following the manufacturer's instructions, add the cajuput essential oil to your diffuser.
2. Hold the diffuser a few inches from your face and inhale through your mouth for 1 minute. Repeat two times daily.

TIP For children under 6 years, replace the cajuput with spearmint essential oil.

Lemon-Mint Vapor

MAKES 1 TREATMENT

2 cups steaming hot (not boiling) water

2 drops lemon essential oil

2 drops peppermint essential oil

1. Pour the water into a shallow bowl and add the lemon and peppermint essential oils.
2. Sitting comfortably in front of the bowl, drape a towel over your head and the bowl, creating a tent that concentrates the steam and vapors. Breathe deeply until the water cools and the vapors subside, emerging for cool air as needed. Repeat once or twice daily.

TIP As an alternative to the vapor tent for children under 12 years, diffuse the essential oils a few feet away from the activity area or in the child's bedroom. A vaporizer or humidifier is another option.

SPLINTER

It's amazing how much pain a tiny sliver of wood can cause when it's lodged in your skin. Instead of trying to dig a stubborn splinter out with a pair of tweezers, coax it out with essential oil. Then, once it's out, stop the pain and prevent infection with these remedies. Lavender, cedarwood, and frankincense are a few good ones to try.

Helichrysum-Chamomile Balm

MAKES ABOUT 1 OUNCE

1 ounce extra-virgin coconut oil, softened

20 drops helichrysum essential oil

10 drops Roman chamomile essential oil

1. In a small jar with a tight-fitting lid, combine the coconut oil with the helichrysum and Roman chamomile essential oils. Stir well with a thin utensil.
2. Carefully remove the splinter and then wash the affected area with soap and water and pat dry.
3. Apply a pea-size amount of the balm to the site, and repeat two to three times daily as needed.

STORAGE Keep in a cool, dark place.

TIP If you don't have helichrysum essential oil, you can replace it with your choice of lavender, frankincense, or myrrh.

Lavender Neat Treatment

MAKES 1 TREATMENT

1 drop lavender essential oil

1. Carefully remove the splinter and then wash the affected area with soap and water and pat dry.
2. Apply the lavender essential oil directly onto the splinter site.

TIP If the splinter is difficult to remove, apply a drop of lavender essential oil to the site and cover it with a bandage. Check the splinter in three to four hours to see if it is ready to come out. Add more lavender if not. Repeat the process until the splinter slides out or dissolves.

Frankincense-Cedarwood Poultice

MAKES 1 TREATMENT

2 drops carrier oil

1 drop frankincense essential oil

1 drop cedarwood essential oil

1. Carefully remove the splinter and then wash the affected area with soap and water and pat dry.
2. Apply the carrier oil and the frankincense and cedarwood essential oils to a cotton ball. Cover the splinter site with the cotton ball, and fasten it in place with an adhesive bandage. Leave until the next bath or shower or until it comes off on its own. If the site is still sore, repeat two or three more times.

TIP If you don't have cedarwood or frankincense essential oil, use cypress or lavender instead.

SPRAIN

Minor sprains and strains lead to pain and swelling that can prevent you from getting around with ease. Be sure to rest the injured site and try to keep the affected limb elevated as much as possible. Combine this care with essential oils—which help by penetrating deep into muscle tissue—and you'll be up and around in no time. Peppermint, pine, and juniper are among the best to try, and they can be used alone or alongside traditional remedies.

Peppermint-Pine Salve

MAKES ABOUT 2 OUNCES

2 ounces extra-virgin coconut oil, softened

16 drops peppermint essential oil

8 drops pine essential oil

1. In a small jar with a tight-fitting lid, combine the coconut oil with the peppermint and pine essential oils. Stir well with a thin utensil.
2. Apply ½ teaspoon of the salve to the affected area, massaging gently. Repeat every two to three hours or as needed.

STORAGE Keep in a cool, dark place.

TIP If you like this balm, you'll be glad to know that it's also useful for a variety of body aches and pains.

Lavender–Tea Tree Balm

MAKES ABOUT ⅓ OUNCE

2 teaspoons safflower oil

20 drops tea tree essential oil

10 drops lavender essential oil

5 drops lemon essential oil

1. In a small bottle with a tight-fitting lid and an orifice reducer, combine the safflower oil with the tea tree, lavender, and lemon essential oils. Secure the lid and shake well to blend.
2. Apply 5 drops of the blend to a cotton ball and swab the affected area, using more if needed. Repeat two to three times daily.

STORAGE Keep in a convenient location if using frequently; otherwise, keep in a cool, dark place.

TIP In a pinch, use either tea tree or lavender essential oil neat; apply 1 or 2 drops to a cotton swab and swab the affected area two to three times daily.

Minty Juniper-Thyme Compress

MAKES ABOUT 2 OUNCES

2 ounces carrier oil

24 drops spearmint essential oil

16 drops juniper essential oil

12 drops thyme essential oil

1. In a small bottle or jar with a tight-fitting lid, combine the carrier oil with the spearmint, juniper, and thyme essential oils. Secure the lid and shake well to blend.
2. Apply 1 teaspoon of the blend to the affected area and cover it with a soft cloth.
3. Place an ice pack over the cloth and leave it in place for 15 to 20 minutes. If the cold becomes uncomfortable, remove it for a minute or two and then reapply. Repeat two to three times daily.

STORAGE Keep in a cool, dark place.

TIP For children under 6 years, omit the juniper essential oil and double the amount of spearmint.

STOMACHACHE

While stomachaches aren't usually serious, the feelings of nausea and discomfort that come with them can interfere with your day's plans or interrupt a good night's sleep. In many cases, essential oils can bring speedy comfort; however, severe stomach pain can be a symptom of something more serious. If your pain persists or worsens, or if your intestinal discomfort is accompanied by a high fever, seek medical treatment right away. →

Ginger-Chamomile Massage Oil

MAKES ABOUT 4 OUNCES

4 ounces carrier oil

20 drops ginger essential oil

10 drops Roman chamomile essential oil

1. In a small bottle or jar with a tight-fitting lid, combine the carrier oil with the ginger and Roman chamomile essential oils. Secure the lid and shake well to blend.
2. Apply 1 teaspoon of the blend to your abdomen and massage gently. Use more if needed, and repeat the treatment two to three times daily.

STORAGE Keep in a cool, dark place.

TIP If you don't have both the ginger and Roman chamomile essential oils on hand, combine 30 drops of either oil with the carrier oil instead.

Vetiver-Ginger Bath Salts

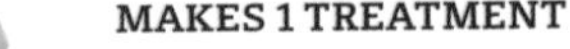

MAKES 1 TREATMENT

1 cup Epsom salt

10 drops ginger essential oil

6 drops vetiver essential oil

1. Draw a warm bath. Add the salt and allow it to dissolve, then add the ginger and vetiver essential oils.
2. Relax in the bath for 15 to 30 minutes.

TIP This relaxing bath-time blend also helps when you're feeling stressed or upset.

Peppermint Stomach Compress

MAKES 1 TREATMENT

1 teaspoon carrier oil

8 drops peppermint essential oil

1. In the palm of your hand, combine the carrier oil with the peppermint essential oil. Rub your hands together briefly and apply the blend to your upper abdomen.
2. Recline comfortably. Cover the essential oil blend with a soft cloth and place a hot pack or heating pad over it. Leave in place for 15 minutes.

TIP For children under 6 years, use spearmint essential oil instead of peppermint.

STREP THROAT

With symptoms that include swelling and bright red tissue with white patches, strep throat brings pain and an unbearable itchy feeling with it. If you think you have strep throat, be sure to see the doctor, since this bacterial infection often requires treatment with antibiotics. While you're using conventional remedies to clear up the infection, you can reach for essential oils that bring relief from the symptoms. Lavender, thyme, and myrrh are among the best. →

Lavender-Thyme Salve

MAKES ABOUT 2 OUNCES

2 ounces extra-virgin coconut oil, softened

16 drops lavender essential oil

16 drops thyme essential oil

1. In a small jar with a tight-fitting lid, combine the coconut oil with the lavender and thyme essential oils. Stir well with a thin utensil.
2. Apply ¼ teaspoon of the salve to your throat, using a little bit more if needed. Repeat every four to six hours or as needed.

STORAGE Keep in a cool, dark place.

TIP If you don't have coconut oil, make this salve using the carrier oil of your choice.

Lemon-Myrrh Throat Spray

MAKES ABOUT 4 OUNCES

4 ounces distilled or purified water

24 drops lemon essential oil

12 drops myrrh essential oil

1. In a small bottle with a fine-mist spray top, combine the water with the lemon and myrrh essential oils and secure the top. Shake well before each use.
2. Open your mouth wide and aim for the back of your throat. Apply one or two spritzes. Repeat three to four times daily.

STORAGE Keep in a cool, dark place.

TIP For young children and those who prefer not to use a throat spray, spritz in the air near your face and take a deep breath through your mouth.

STRESS

With all the demands on our busy lives, it's sometimes hard to imagine a day without stress. No one is immune to this condition, but that doesn't mean we should just grin and bear it. If you are feeling the effects of stress, essential oils can help you relax and unwind. Vetiver, lavender, bergamot, and ylang-ylang balance turbulent emotions and act as sedatives, but without any undesirable side effects.

Clary Sage–Mandarin Diffusion

MAKES 1 TREATMENT

2 drops mandarin essential oil

1 drop clary sage essential oil

Following the manufacturer's instructions, add the mandarin and clary sage essential oils to your diffuser. Run the diffuser nearby. Repeat every two to three hours or as needed.

TIP This is a fantastic blend for vapor therapy, too. Use it in a humidifier or vaporizer, or add the essential oils to your bath.

Bergamot-Chamomile Aromatic Spray

MAKES ABOUT 4 OUNCES

4 ounces distilled or purified water

20 drops bergamot essential oil

20 drops chamomile essential oil

1. In a small bottle with a fine-mist spray top, combine the water with the bergamot and chamomile essential oils and secure the top. Shake well before each use.
2. Spritz clothing or upholstery a few times.

STORAGE Keep in a cool, dark place.

TIP Create a blend for diffusion by combining the bergamot and chamomile essential oils in a small bottle with a tight-fitting lid and an orifice reducer. Secure the lid and shake well to blend. Diffuse 2 or 3 drops in the room where you spend the most time.

Ylang-Ylang Neat Treatment

MAKES 1 TREATMENT

2 drops ylang-ylang essential oil

Apply the ylang-ylang essential oil directly to your temples or to your inner wrists and neck. Breathe deeply and relax for a few minutes.

TIP Relax and unwind by adding 3 or 4 drops of ylang-ylang essential oil to a warm bath.

STRETCH MARKS

These discolored streaks or stripes on your skin don't cause you any physical pain, but they can make you feel self-conscious. You might even avoid wearing certain styles of clothing to keep them hidden. Essential oils don't work overnight, but with time and consistent use, they can help fade the unwanted marks. Whenever possible, apply the remedy as soon as you notice stretch marks developing. If that happens to be during pregnancy, replace the essential oils in these recipes with an equal amount of lavender essential oil only, to prevent sensitivity.

Lavender-Geranium Massage Oil

MAKES ABOUT 4 OUNCES

4 ounces extra-virgin coconut oil, softened

20 drops lavender essential oil

15 drops geranium essential oil

1. In a small jar with a tight-fitting lid, combine the coconut oil with the lavender and geranium essential oils. Stir well with a thin utensil.
2. After showering, apply a pea-size amount of the blend to each area where stretch marks are present, using a little more if needed. Repeat once or twice daily.

STORAGE Keep in a convenient location if using frequently; otherwise, keep in a cool, dark place.

TIP This blend is also useful for dry skin. Try it on problem areas like knees, elbows, and heels.

Mandarin-Vetiver Cream

MAKES ABOUT 4 OUNCES

4 ounces cocoa butter

20 drops mandarin essential oil

12 drops vetiver essential oil

1. In a small jar with a tight-fitting lid, combine the cocoa butter with the mandarin and vetiver essential oils. Stir well with a thin utensil.
2. Apply ½ teaspoon of the blend in a thin layer to each affected area, using a little more or less as needed. Repeat once or twice daily.

STORAGE Keep in a cool, dark place.

TIP For a non-photosensitizing cream, replace the mandarin essential oil with an equal amount of patchouli or helichrysum.

Helichrysum Neat Treatment

MAKES 1 TREATMENT

1 drop helichrysum essential oil (per area)

Apply the helichrysum essential oil directly to each affected area. Repeat once daily.

TIP This helichrysum neat treatment helps reduce the appearance of scars, too.

STUFFY NOSE

Whether a stuffy nose accompanies the flu, a cold, or allergies, essential oils can help you breathe easier, faster. Eucalyptus is my go-to for clearing up a stuffy nose, but there are many others that can help, too. Among the best are tea tree, lavender, rosemary, and mint. Other helpful oils include those in the citrus family, such as lemon, mandarin, and grapefruit.

Peppermint-Lavender Vapor

MAKES 1 TREATMENT

2 cups steaming hot (not boiling) water

2 drops peppermint essential oil

2 drops lavender essential oil

1. Pour the water into a shallow bowl and add the lavender and peppermint essential oils.
2. Sitting comfortably in front of the bowl, drape a towel over your head and the bowl, creating a tent that concentrates the steam and vapors. Breathe deeply until the water cools and the vapors subside, emerging for cool air as needed. Repeat once or twice daily.

TIP If you have time, apply the peppermint and lavender essential oils to a washcloth and take it into the shower, placing it opposite the showerhead, or add them to your bathwater.

Eucalyptus Diffusion

MAKES 1 TREATMENT

2 drops eucalyptus essential oil

Following the manufacturer's instructions, add the eucalyptus essential oil to your diffuser. Run the diffuser nearby. Repeat once or twice daily.

TIP Eucalyptus has a strong smell in the bottle, but diffusing it in your home lends a fresh, clean fragrance. Use it to banish strong odors and kill airborne bacteria.

Lemony Lavender-Rosemary Balm

MAKES ABOUT 1 OUNCE

1 ounce jojoba oil

16 drops rosemary essential oil

10 drops lemon essential oil

10 drops lavender essential oil

1. In a small bottle or jar with a tight-fitting lid, combine the jojoba oil with the rosemary, lemon, and lavender essential oils. Secure the lid and shake well to blend.
2. Apply ¼ to ½ teaspoon of the balm to a cotton ball and swab your forehead, cheekbones, and throat. Repeat each evening at bedtime.

STORAGE Keep in a cool, dark place.

TIP This balm has a refreshing fragrance, plus it can help heal cracked skin. Use it on painful cuticles, dry elbows and knees, and other problem areas.

STY

Sties are rarely serious, but the irritation and swelling can make you very uncomfortable. Most of the time, a sty will pop up on the edge of the eyelid, usually beginning when bacteria invades the root of an eyelash. Antibacterial essential oils target the bacteria, preventing the inflammation and swelling from worsening. Since even mild essential oils can burn delicate tissue, essential oils are never directly applied to the eye.

Lavender Neat Treatment

MAKES 1 TREATMENT

1 drop lavender essential oil

Apply the lavender essential oil directly to your cheekbone, about 1 inch beneath the affected eye. Repeat twice daily.

TIP For children younger than 6 years, dilute 1 drop of lavender essential oil in 4 drops of carrier oil, and apply 1 drop of the dilution to the cheekbone as described.

Chamomile Compress

MAKES 1 TREATMENT

4 drops distilled or purified water

1 drop Roman chamomile essential oil

1. Apply the water and Roman chamomile essential oil to a cotton ball. Lie down and close the affected eye. →

Chamomile Compress continued

2. Gently press the cotton ball onto your eye. Leave it in place for 10 to 15 minutes while you relax. Repeat twice daily or more often as needed to ease discomfort.

TIP This compress also helps swollen, inflamed pimples heal faster and can be used on small areas of inflamed skin.

SUNBURN

Depending on the day and time of year, just a little time out in the sun without sun protection can cause a burn. And even when you try to remember to keep applying your sunscreen, it isn't unheard of to get sunburn after a day of hiking or on the beach. Essential oils can help ease the sting of a fresh sunburn, plus they can help compromised tissue heal faster. If you can't reach all the sunburned areas on your body, you may want to get a helper to give you a hand with application.

Cooling Spearmint-Lavender Gel

MAKES ABOUT 4 OUNCES

4 ounces aloe vera gel

20 drops lavender essential oil

10 drops spearmint essential oil

1. In a small jar with a tight-fitting lid, combine the aloe gel with the lavender and spearmint essential oils. Stir well with a thin utensil.
2. Apply 1 teaspoon of the gel to the sunburn, using more or less to create a thin layer. Allow the skin to dry before dressing. Repeat as needed to relieve discomfort.

STORAGE Keep in a cool, dark place or store in the refrigerator for a cooling sensation with each use.

TIP You can also use this remedy to ease congestion by applying ½ teaspoon of the gel to your chest and neck area.

Chamomile–Tea Tree Spray

MAKES ABOUT 8 OUNCES

8 ounces alcohol-free witch hazel

20 drops Roman chamomile essential oil

10 drops tea tree essential oil

1. In a small bottle with a fine-mist spray top, combine the witch hazel with the Roman chamomile and tea tree essential oils. Secure the top and shake well to blend.
2. Spray generously onto sunburned areas. Allow the skin to dry before dressing. Repeat as needed to relieve discomfort.

STORAGE Keep in a cool, dark place.

TIP This spray makes a great anti-itch therapy for eczema, too.

Lavender-Helichrysum Salve

MAKES ABOUT 4 OUNCES

4 ounces extra-virgin coconut oil, softened

40 drops lavender essential oil

20 drops helichrysum essential oil

1. In a small jar with a tight-fitting lid, combine the coconut oil with the lavender and helichrysum essential oils. Stir with a thin utensil.
2. Apply ½ teaspoon of the blend to the palm of your hand and allow it to melt. Gently apply a thin layer to burned areas, using more if needed. Repeat two to three times daily.

STORAGE Keep in a cool, dark place.

TIP If you prefer a lighter blend, you can replace the coconut oil with aloe vera gel.

SWIMMER'S EAR

When water gets trapped in your ears, the warmth, darkness, and moisture create the perfect environment for bacteria to grow. Essential oils can bring relief from discomfort while killing the bacteria. When you use these remedies as soon as you notice a little bit of tickling or itching in your ear, you'll prevent the problem from getting worse. Since bacteria can spread, be sure to treat both ears even if only one seems to be affected.

Eucalyptus Neat Treatment

MAKES 1 TREATMENT

4 drops eucalyptus essential oil

Apply the eucalyptus essential oil directly, starting behind each ear and working toward the corner of the jaw and down the side of the throat, all the way to the chest. Repeat twice daily.

TIP For children under 6 years, replace the eucalyptus essential oil with lavender.

Lavender-Rosemary Compress

MAKES 1 TREATMENT

4 drops lavender essential oil

4 drops rosemary essential oil

1. Apply 2 drops of lavender and 2 drops of rosemary essential oil to each of two cotton balls.
2. Tuck one cotton ball into each ear. Relax for 15 to 30 minutes. Repeat two to three times daily.

TIP This remedy is also ideal for other types of earaches and ear infections.

SWOLLEN ANKLES OR FEET

Long hours spent standing in one place can cause feet and ankles to swell, and so can sitting for hours on end. Shoes start to feel tight, and sometimes the swelling is so bad that it's painful to put your shoes back on once you've taken them off. Diuretic essential oils can speed relief by encouraging swollen tissues to release excess water, and by soothing the tight, uncomfortable feeling that affects the skin, muscles, and joints.

Peppermint-Lemon Salt Scrub

MAKES ABOUT 8 OUNCES

6 ounces Epsom salt

2 ounces carrier oil

30 drops lemon essential oil

15 drops peppermint essential oil

1. In a small jar with a tight-fitting lid, combine the salt and carrier oil with the lemon and peppermint essential oils. Secure the lid and shake well to blend.
2. While bathing or showering, use 1 teaspoon of the scrub to thoroughly massage your feet. Repeat every two to three days.

STORAGE Keep in a cool, dark place.

TIP This remedy is good for exfoliating and moisturizing dry skin on hands, elbows, knees, and other problem areas, too.

Grapefruit Massage Cream

MAKES ABOUT 8 OUNCES

8 ounces cocoa butter

1 teaspoon grapefruit essential oil

1. In a small jar with a tight-fitting lid, combine the cocoa butter with the grapefruit essential oil. Stir well with a thin utensil.
2. Apply ¼ teaspoon of the massage cream to each foot, massaging gently and working your way up the calf, using more cream if needed. Repeat once or twice daily.

STORAGE Keep in a cool, dark place.

TIP This cream also helps reduce the appearance of stretch marks and cellulite. For those issues, use it daily.

Minty Citrus-Thyme Balm

MAKES ABOUT 4 OUNCES

4 ounces aloe vera gel

20 drops grapefruit essential oil

20 drops mandarin essential oil

10 drops spearmint essential oil

10 drops thyme essential oil →

Minty Citrus-Thyme Balm continued

1. In a small jar with a tight-fitting lid, combine the aloe gel with the grapefruit, mandarin, spearmint, and thyme essential oils. Stir well with a thin utensil.
2. Apply ½ teaspoon of the balm to each affected foot or ankle. Use more if needed and repeat the treatment two to three times daily.

STORAGE Keep in a cool, dark place.

TIP This refreshing blend is ideal for soothing tired legs after a long day. It's even nicer when kept cool in the refrigerator.

TEETH GRINDING

If teeth grinding goes on long enough, jaw disorders, tooth damage, and headaches can result. This disorder involves unconscious sleep-related movements, and it often goes unnoticed until discomfort sets in. Some symptoms include jaw and/or facial pain, earache-type pain, or damage to the insides of your cheeks. Seek dental care for damaged teeth, and address sources of stress, which may be a contributing factor. Reach for sedative essential oils while you're getting to the root of the problem; they can help you relax and grind less. While you're at it, consider using analgesic oils to deal with sore muscles and other symptoms.

Lavender Neat Treatment

MAKES 1 TREATMENT

6 to 8 drops lavender essential oil

Apply lavender essential oil directly to the sole of each foot before bed. Focus on relaxing as you drift off to sleep.

TIP Use this treatment anytime tension or stress threatens peaceful sleep.

Chamomile, Orange, and Ylang-Ylang Diffusion

MAKES 1 TREATMENT

3 drops Roman chamomile essential oil

3 drops sweet orange essential oil

2 drops ylang-ylang essential oil

Following the manufacturer's instructions, add the Roman chamomile, sweet orange, and ylang-ylang essential oils to your diffuser. Run the diffuser in your bedroom before turning in for the night. Repeat nightly.

TIP If you don't have ylang-ylang essential oil, you can replace it with 4 drops of lavender.

TENDINITIS

Tendinitis is often a repetitive-motion injury, occurring when you move a specific body part in a certain way, over and over again. The pain you feel is caused by inflammation, and in serious cases, surgical intervention is the only way to get relief. Luckily, if your tendinitis is the result of too much smartphone or tablet use, overexertion on the tennis court, or typing for hours on end, essential oils can bring some relief. Try to reduce or stop the repetitive activities that led to the problem in the first place, since continuing the activity will only make your tendinitis worse.

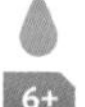

6+

Juniper-Peppermint Salve

MAKES ABOUT 4 OUNCES

4 ounces extra-virgin coconut oil, softened

20 drops juniper essential oil

20 drops peppermint essential oil

1. In a small jar with a tight-fitting lid, combine the coconut oil with the juniper and peppermint essential oils. Stir with a thin utensil.
2. Apply ¼ teaspoon of the salve to the affected area, using a little more or less as needed. Repeat two to three times daily.

STORAGE Keep in a cool, dark place.

TIP If you prefer a lighter blend, you can replace the coconut oil with aloe vera gel.

Helichrysum-Thyme Compress

MAKES 1 TREATMENT

4 drops carrier oil

4 drops helichrysum essential oil

4 drops thyme essential oil

1. In a small bowl, combine the carrier oil with the helichrysum and thyme essential oils.
2. Dip a cotton ball into the blend until it is completely absorbed, swab the blend over the affected area, and cover it with a towel.
3. Apply a warm heating pad and leave it in place for 10 to 15 minutes. Repeat every two to three hours or as needed.

TIP If you don't have time for a compress, you can simply apply the blend as a muscle rub.

Peppermint Neat Treatment

MAKES 1 TREATMENT

3 or 4 drops peppermint essential oil

Apply the peppermint essential oil to a cotton pad and swab the painful area. Repeat every four to five hours, or as often as needed.

TIP If treating someone who is pregnant or under 6 years, use spearmint essential oil instead of peppermint.

THRUSH

Oral thrush is caused by Candida albicans, *a type of yeast that can wreak havoc on your entire system. Thrush often begins as a few painless white patches inside the mouth, but these can quickly grow larger and become inflamed. Red, angry lesions often erupt, too, and in some cases, the corners of the mouth may crack and bleed. Antifungal essential oils can be a tremendous help, and if you address the problem early enough, they can eliminate symptoms very quickly.*

Lavender Salve

MAKES 1 TREATMENT

6 drops extra-virgin olive oil

1 drop lavender essential oil

1. In a small bowl, combine the olive oil with the lavender essential oil. Stir with a thin utensil.
2. Saturate a cotton ball in the blend until it is completely absorbed, and gently swab the salve onto the lesions.
3. Breathe through your mouth for two minutes to give the treatment as much time to penetrate as possible. Repeat twice daily.

TIP If thrush has spread from an affected baby's mouth to a nursing mom's nipple, apply lavender oil neat to the area. It's fine for the baby to nurse once the essential oil has been absorbed.

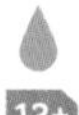

Lemon-Thyme Oil-Pulling Treatment

12+

MAKES 1 TREATMENT

½ tablespoon extra-virgin olive oil

1 drop lemon essential oil

1 drop thyme essential oil

1. In a shot glass, combine the olive oil with the lemon and thyme essential oils, and stir with a thin utensil.
2. Pour the liquid into your mouth and swish the oil across your teeth and gums.
3. When you have coated all the surfaces of your mouth, spit the oil into a paper towel and discard.
4. Wait 5 minutes and then rinse your mouth with water. Repeat once daily.

TIP If you are missing either the lemon or thyme essential oil, use lavender as a replacement.

VOMITING

As disgusting and uncomfortable as it may be, vomiting is one of the body's best defenses against toxins. Essential oils can help you feel better after vomiting, and their antispasmodic actions can sometimes help prevent you from enduring wave after wave of nausea. Try these treatments if you're suffering from the flu or food poisoning, and give them a go if you've got a nasty hangover. If vomiting is accompanied by a high fever or you're throwing up blood, seek emergency medical treatment. →

Ginger Ear Massage Oil

MAKES 1 TREATMENT

3 drops carrier oil

3 drops ginger essential oil

In the palm of your hand, combine the carrier oil with the ginger essential oil. Rub your hands together briefly and then apply the blend to the backside of each ear and breathe deeply. Repeat every two to three hours or as needed.

TIP If you don't have ginger essential oil, try this treatment with peppermint or spearmint instead.

Peppermint Vapor

MAKES 1 TREATMENT

2 drops peppermint essential oil

1 cup steaming hot (not boiling) water

1. Add the peppermint essential oil directly to the cup of water and breathe in the vapors.
2. Keep the cup with you until the fragrance subsides. Repeat as often as needed.

TIP Peppermint can also be used neat by applying 1 drop to each temple. Relax and focus on taking deep, calming breaths. Replace the peppermint essential oil with spearmint if you are pregnant or treating a child under 6 years.

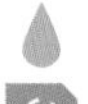
6+

Chamomile-Peppermint Massage Oil

MAKES 1 TREATMENT

4 drops carrier oil

6 drops peppermint essential oil

4 drops Roman chamomile essential oil

In the palm of your hand, combine the carrier oil with the peppermint and Roman chamomile essential oils. Rub your hands together briefly and then apply the blend to your upper abdomen, focusing on the area just below your sternum. Repeat once or twice daily while symptoms persist.

TIP Treat children under 6 years by replacing the peppermint essential oil with spearmint.

WATER RETENTION

Often the result of monthly hormone shifts or eating too many salty snacks, water retention leads to unpleasant swelling and weight gain. Luckily, diuretic essential oils can help your body get rid of the excess water and return to its normal size. If you tend to retain fluid frequently and you don't think salt or your monthly cycle is to blame, see your doctor. Chronic water retention can be a sign of serious illness, including kidney or liver disease. →

Grapefruit Massage Oil

MAKES ABOUT 4 OUNCES

4 ounces jojoba oil

24 drops grapefruit essential oil

1. In a small jar with a tight-fitting lid, combine the jojoba oil with the grapefruit essential oil. Secure the lid and shake well to blend.
2. Apply 1 teaspoon of the blend to your abdomen, adding more if needed. Massage gently for 5 minutes. Repeat once or twice daily.

STORAGE Keep in a cool, dark place.

TIP Use this blend on your temples anytime you're feeling zapped or out of sorts. The uplifting fragrance will improve your mood quickly.

Cypress-Geranium Bath Salts

MAKES ABOUT 16 OUNCES

2 cups Epsom salt

1 tablespoon carrier oil

20 drops cypress essential oil

20 drops geranium essential oil

1. In a quart jar with a tight-fitting lid, combine the salt and carrier oil with the cypress and geranium essential oils. Secure the lid and shake well to blend.

2. Draw a warm bath. Add ½ cup of the bath salts and allow them to dissolve. Soak for 15 to 30 minutes. Repeat daily or use as needed.

STORAGE Keep in a cool, dark place.

TIP These bath salts are ideal for treating stress and anxiety, too.

Citrus-Thyme Lotion

MAKES ABOUT 8 OUNCES

8 ounces unscented body lotion

20 drops grapefruit essential oil

10 drops lemon essential oil

10 drops mandarin essential oil

10 drops thyme essential oil

1. In a small jar with a tight-fitting lid, combine the body lotion with the grapefruit, lemon, mandarin, and thyme essential oils. Secure the lid and shake well to combine.
2. Apply 1 teaspoon of the blend to your entire body, using more or less as needed. Repeat two or three times daily.

STORAGE Keep in a cool, dark place.

TIP This uplifting blend also helps improve a dark mood. Apply a small amount to your hands anytime you need a quick boost.

YEAST INFECTION

Itching, soreness, and discharge make yeast infections one of the most uncomfortable maladies. Due to an overgrowth of Candida albicans, *which occurs naturally in the body and rarely causes problems, yeast infections are seldom serious enough to require medical intervention. Essential oil treatments are admittedly earthy, but they bring quick relief. You can find douche syringes online and in well-stocked drugstores.*

Myrrh Poultice

MAKES 1 TREATMENT

1 teaspoon extra-virgin coconut oil, softened

3 drops myrrh essential oil

1. In a small bowl, combine the coconut oil with the myrrh essential oil. Mix well with a thin utensil.
2. Coat an applicator-free tampon with the blend.
3. Insert the coated tampon into the vagina. Leave the tampon in place for one to two hours. Repeat the treatment two or three times daily until symptoms subside.

TIP If you don't have myrrh, use lavender or tea tree essential oil instead.

Tea Tree Douche

MAKES ABOUT 16 OUNCES

8 ounces distilled or purified water

8 ounces alcohol-free witch hazel

16 drops tea tree essential oil

1. In a quart jar with a tight-fitting lid, combine the water and witch hazel with the tea tree essential oil. Secure the lid and shake well.
2. Draw 2 ounces of the solution into the douche syringe.
3. Use the syringe in the shower according to the manufacturer's recommendations. Repeat once or twice daily until symptoms are gone.

STORAGE Keep in a cool, dark place.

TIP If you don't have witch hazel, replace it with the same amount of additional distilled or purified water and increase to 20 drops of tea tree essential oil.

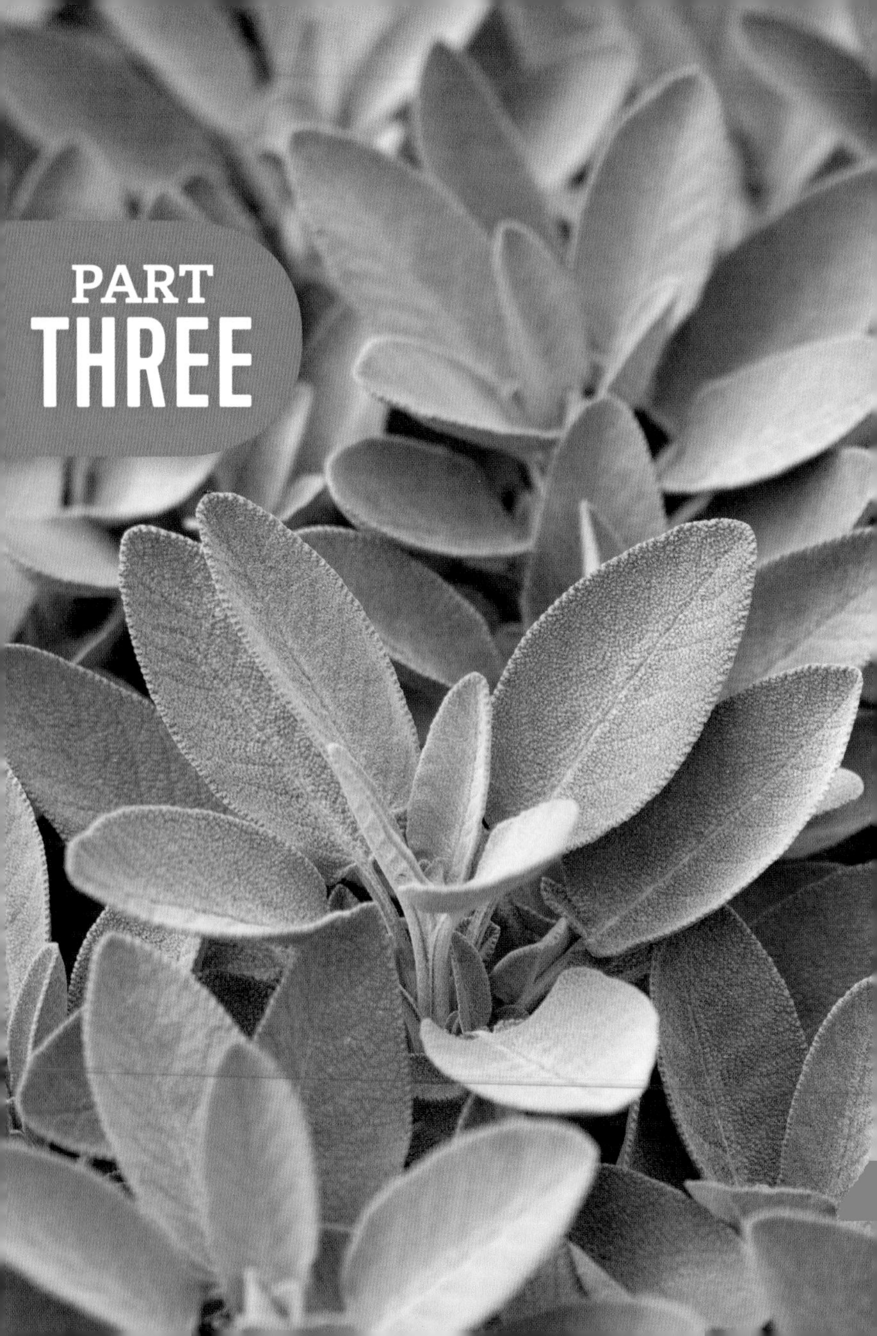

PART THREE

50 Essential Oils in Profile

Once you start using essential oils, you might find yourself discovering more and more ways to enjoy them. After all, why waste money on chemical cleansers for your home when essential oils smell better and work just as well, and why run the risk of unwanted side effects by taking OTC painkillers when something as simple as peppermint can bring fast, effective relief from a headache?

Before you jump in with both feet though, it's a good idea to take some time to familiarize yourself with the essential oils you'd like to use. There are hundreds to choose from, but most people work from a relatively compact arsenal that typically starts with very common oils like lavender, tea tree, peppermint or spearmint, or eucalyptus.

This part contains short profiles in a user-friendly format that's easy to refer to when you're shopping for oils or looking for a way to address an ailment. Begin by accessing the Latin name for the essential oil you're considering, and use that information as a starting point to confirm that the essential oils in your shopping cart are derived from the species described here. Knowing Latin names might seem like overkill, but labels can be confusing.

Taking a moment to double-check is your key to finding exactly what you want and feeling confident enough to use it.

As you'll soon discover, each of the essential oils outlined in this section has a multitude of uses, blends well with others in terms of fragrance and effectiveness, and offers specific medicinal properties that make it well suited for a variety of ailments. You can find a glossary of medicinal properties starting on page 287.

Most essential oils come with a few precautions, too. These aren't meant to scare you but to remind you that plant constituents are powerful medicine indeed. In some people, such as young children and pregnant women, the use of certain oils can cause undesirable consequences. In these and other cases, it's best to err on the side of caution if you're not certain about an essential oil. If you're planning to spend time outdoors, you might opt to skip an essential oil that cautions you to avoid sunlight, and choose a different one.

As you learn more about essential oils, you'll find that the Internet is a great resource. At the same time, there's a lot of conflicting information to wade through. These profiles offer a time-saving solution by serving as a handy reference to the essential oils you're likely to find yourself buying and using most frequently.

ANISE

Pimpinella anisum

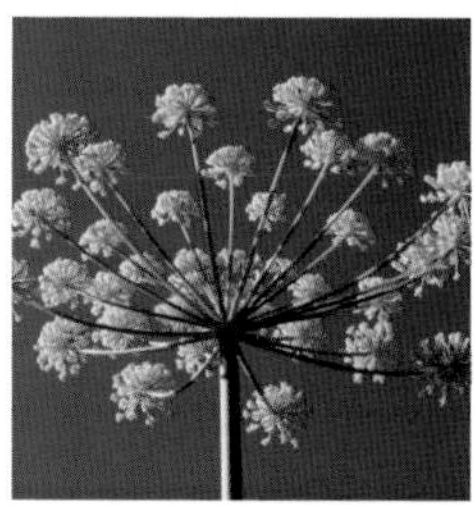

Sometimes referred to as aniseed or anise seed, this essential oil offers an enticing licorice aroma. If anise sounds familiar to you, it's because this essential oil comes from a very popular herb used primarily in Indian and Turkish cuisine. Anise essential oil is an excellent remedy for nausea, vomiting, and other digestive complaints. Diffuse two or three drops to experience fast relief.

BLENDS WELL WITH

cedarwood, dill, ginger, mandarin, pine, rose, sweet orange

CAN BE SUBSTITUTED WITH

fennel, ginger

PRECAUTIONS

Avoid use with children 6 years or younger; Not recommended for use during pregnancy; Avoid use if suffering from an estrogen-dependent cancer; May cause skin irritation

MEDICINAL PROPERTIES

analgesic, anti-anxiety, antiseptic, antispasmodic, digestive, diuretic, expectorant

IDEAL FOR TREATING

allergies, anxiety, asthma, bronchitis, cough, eczema, fever, insect bites, minor wounds, sunburn

BASIL

Ocimum basilicum

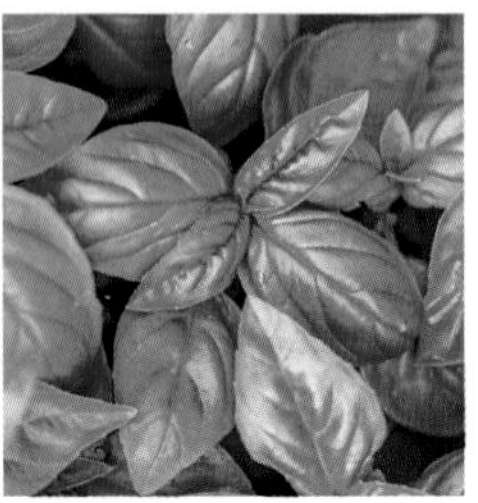

With an energizing fragrance that many find intoxicating, basil essential oil is an excellent choice for relieving exhaustion. Besides its ability to improve your mental state when you're feeling foggy, it stimulates circulation, helping ease pain and speed the healing process. Try basil for tension headaches, muscle pain, and stiff joints. It's also an excellent addition to cold and flu remedies.

BLENDS WELL WITH

bergamot, cedarwood, citronella, clary sage, ginger, lemon, rosemary, sweet orange

CAN BE SUBSTITUTED WITH

fir needle, juniper, pine

PRECAUTIONS

Avoid use with children 12 years or younger; Avoid use if pregnant; Avoid use if suffering from epilepsy; May cause skin irritation

MEDICINAL PROPERTIES

analgesic, anti-inflammatory, antiseptic, digestive, emmenagogue, expectorant, stimulant

IDEAL FOR TREATING

anxiety, colic, cough, cramping, hangover, indigestion, menstrual discomfort, muscle aches, nausea, vertigo

BENZOIN

Styrax benzoin

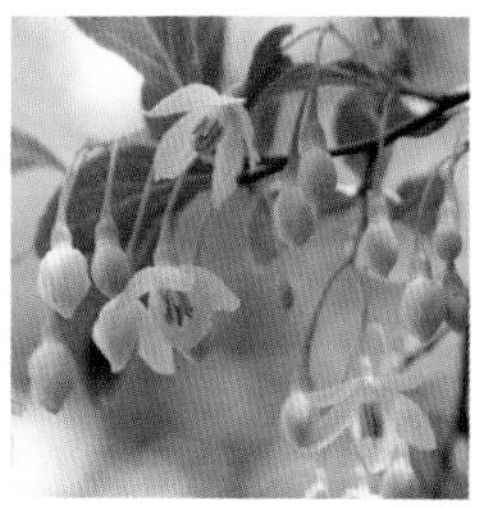

While you may not have heard of benzoin, it's likely you've smelled a hint of its warm, sweet fragrance. A favorite in the perfume industry, this oil is also used by incense manufacturers. Benzoin is one of my favorite remedies for dealing with stress; like frankincense and myrrh, it promotes a sense of peaceful well-being. It's also great for skin. Try it for acne, rashes, or fading scar tissue.

BLENDS WELL WITH

bergamot, fir needle, frankincense, juniper, myrrh, rose, sweet orange

CAN BE SUBSTITUTED WITH

hyssop, lavandin, spike lavender

PRECAUTIONS

Avoid use with children 6 years or younger; Avoid use before driving or operating machinery

MEDICINAL PROPERTIES

antidepressant, anti-inflammatory, antiseptic, diuretic, expectorant, sedative, vulnerary

IDEAL FOR TREATING

acne, bronchitis, cold, cough, eczema, insomnia, muscle pain, muscle stiffness, stress, water retention

BERGAMOT

Citrus bergamia

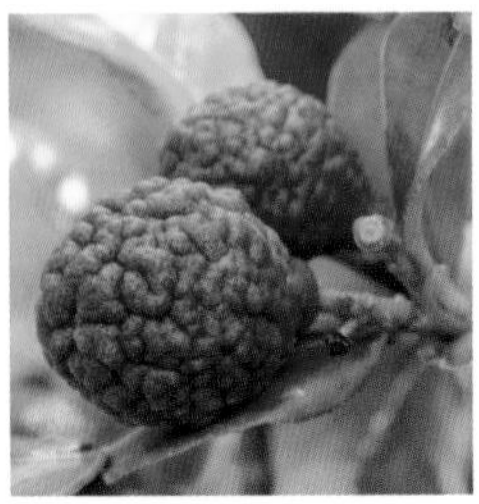

With an irresistible aroma that uplifts your spirits almost instantly, bergamot essential oil gives Earl Grey tea its signature scent. It is also a favorite perfume ingredient. Made from the unripe fruit of a small citrus tree, it has a light texture and a pale green to greenish-yellow color. Bergamot's antiseptic property makes it useful for treating skin problems, and its uplifting fragrance can help you cope with mild depression, grief, and seasonal affective disorder (SAD).

BLENDS WELL WITH

clary sage, frankincense, mandarin

CAN BE SUBSTITUTED WITH

grapefruit, lemon, lime, mandarin

PRECAUTIONS

Avoid sunlight after use; Avoid use with children 6 years or younger; May cause skin irritation

MEDICINAL PROPERTIES

analgesic, antibacterial, antidepressant, antiseptic, calmative, digestive, febrifuge

IDEAL FOR TREATING

acne, chicken pox, cold, eczema, flu, mild depression, postpartum depression, psoriasis, stress, urinary tract infection

CAJUPUT

Melaleuca cajuputi

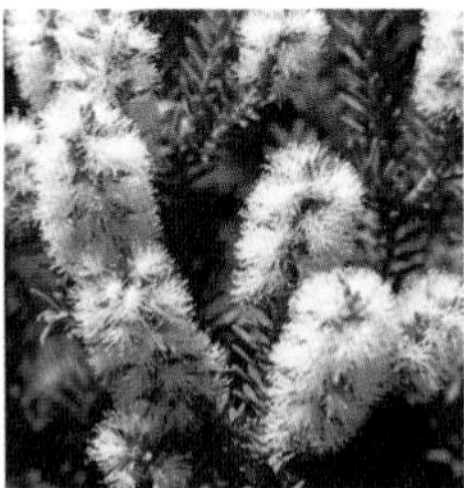

Also known as cajeput or white tea tree essential oil, this extract is best known for its antiseptic properties. In India and Malaysia, where the trees grow wild, it is used as a traditional remedy for a variety of illnesses, including upset stomach and cholera. It is also used as a natural insecticide. Besides calming the digestive system, cajuput can help ease body aches, earaches, headaches, and many other painful conditions.

BLENDS WELL WITH

bergamot, cypress, eucalyptus, juniper, pine

CAN BE SUBSTITUTED WITH

tea tree, white camphor

PRECAUTIONS

Avoid use with children 6 years or younger; May cause skin irritation; May irritate mucous membranes

MEDICINAL PROPERTIES

analgesic, antiseptic, antispasmodic, decongestant, expectorant, febrifuge, insecticidal, stimulant

IDEAL FOR TREATING

asthma, bronchitis, cold, cough, headache, nausea, oily skin, psoriasis, sinusitis, sore throat

CARROT SEED

Daucus carota

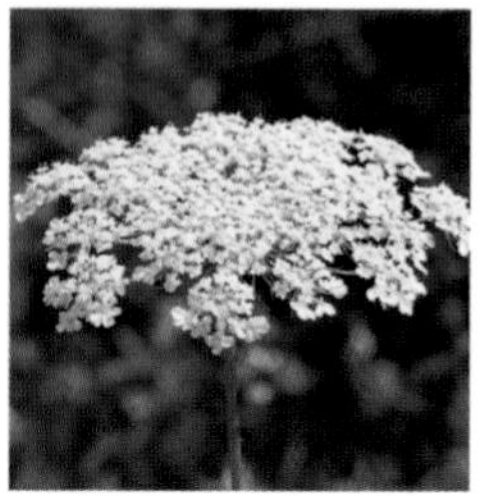

Carrot seed essential oil comes from wild carrot plants rather than the domesticated kind that make their way into your salad. Thanks to its healing and stimulating properties, this lightly fragrant essential oil is among the best for dealing with problem skin. It's an excellent detoxifier and diuretic, too, making it a good choice for dealing with water retention and hangovers.

BLENDS WELL WITH

bergamot, cedarwood, cinnamon bark, ginger, lemon, nutmeg, rose geranium

CAN BE SUBSTITUTED WITH

geranium, grapefruit, rose geranium

PRECAUTIONS

Generally considered safe

MEDICINAL PROPERTIES

analgesic, antiseptic, carminative, detoxifying, diuretic, stimulant

IDEAL FOR TREATING

bronchitis, cuts and scrapes, dermatitis, eczema, edema, flu, muscle aches, rashes, stress, water retention

CATNIP

Nepeta cataria

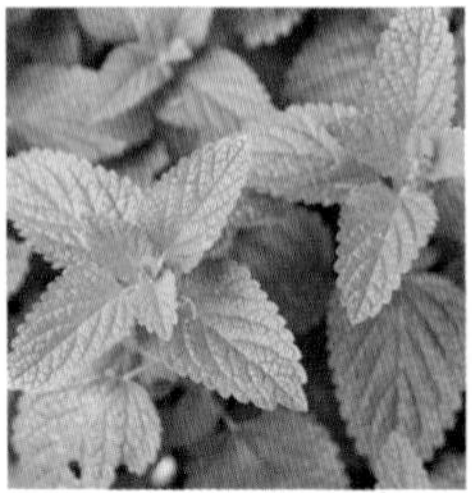

Offering a complex, herbaceous aroma that many people appreciate, catnip essential oil is an outstanding insect repellent, even when used in very small amounts. When diffused, it acts as a sedative and stress reliever, and when applied to cat toys, it makes feline playtime more fun. Catnip's anti-inflammatory action makes it useful for easing joint and muscle pain.

BLENDS WELL WITH

cedarwood, citronella, geranium, lemongrass, peppermint, rose geranium, spearmint

CAN BE SUBSTITUTED WITH

citronella, lemongrass, rose geranium

PRECAUTIONS

Avoid use if pregnant; Avoid use before driving or operating machinery; May cause skin irritation

MEDICINAL PROPERTIES

anti-inflammatory, antispasmodic, astringent, digestive, febrifuge, sedative

IDEAL FOR TREATING

anxiety, headache, indigestion, insomnia, nervousness, stress

CEDARWOOD

Juniperus virginiana

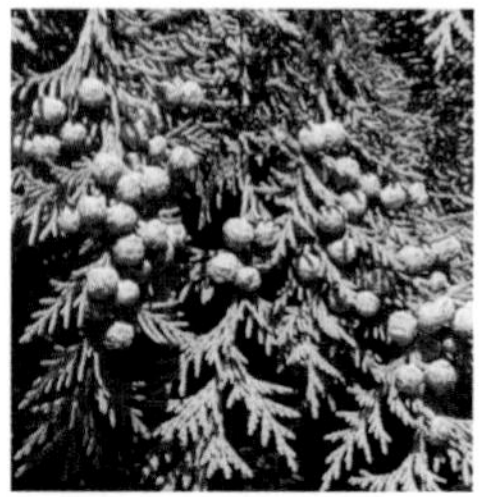

With a soft, woody fragrance that most people find irresistible, cedarwood essential oil has a pale yellow color and a viscous texture. Its aroma offers a calming property that can help balance your emotions, and its expectorant property makes it an excellent choice for use in cough and cold remedies. As an astringent, cedarwood is ideal for itchy, irritating skin conditions ranging from acne to dandruff.

BLENDS WELL WITH

bergamot, cypress, frankincense

CAN BE SUBSTITUTED WITH

cypress, juniper, lemon, rosemary, sandalwood

PRECAUTIONS

Avoid use with children 6 years or younger; Avoid use if pregnant; May cause skin irritation

MEDICINAL PROPERTIES

antifungal, antiseborrheic, antiseptic, antispasmodic, astringent, diuretic, emmenagogue, expectorant

IDEAL FOR TREATING

acne, anxiety, bronchitis, cold, cough, dandruff, nervousness, psoriasis, urinary tract infection

CINNAMON BARK

Cinnamomum verum

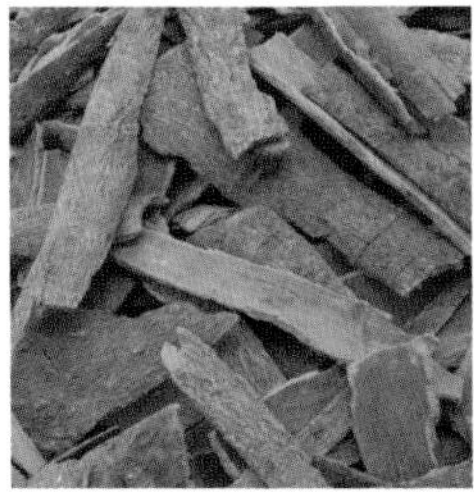

Like the familiar spice, cinnamon bark essential oil has a lovely fragrance. Its warming property brings quick relief to stiff or sore muscles, and it's a good one to diffuse when you're suffering from an upper respiratory illness. Cinnamon bark essential oil is ideal for natural insect control, and it's my go-to for eliminating odors in the kitchen garbage disposal. Add a few drops at night, and you'll wake up to a fresh-smelling kitchen.

BLENDS WELL WITH

benzoin, clove, frankincense, ginger, lemon, rose, ylang-ylang

CAN BE SUBSTITUTED WITH

clove, ginger, nutmeg

PRECAUTIONS

Avoid use with children 6 years or younger; Avoid use if pregnant; Avoid contact with mucous membranes; Dilute well before use

MEDICINAL PROPERTIES

analgesic, antibacterial, antidepressant, antiseptic, aphrodisiac, emmenagogue, insecticidal

IDEAL FOR TREATING

bronchitis, cold, cough, depression, flu, muscle cramps, muscle soreness, painful periods

CITRONELLA

Cymbopogon nardus, Andropogon nardus

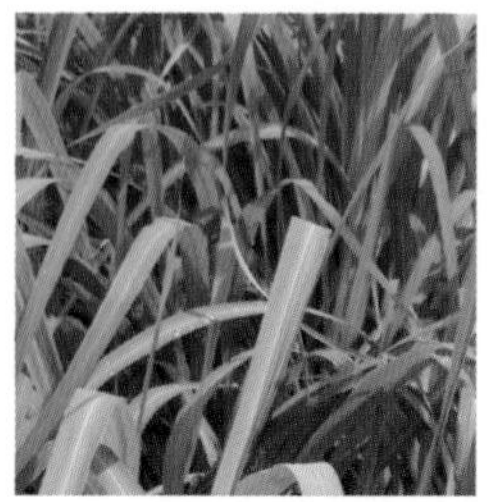

It's quite likely that you've smelled the aroma of citronella. This powerful essential oil is an excellent one for keeping mosquitos and gnats from spoiling outdoor fun, and it's a common ingredient in commercial bug sprays. When you purchase citronella essential oil, make sure you're getting the real thing and not a paraffin- or mineral-oil-based product.

BLENDS WELL WITH

bergamot, cedarwood, lavender, lemon, oregano, pine, rose geranium

CAN BE SUBSTITUTED WITH

catnip, geranium, lemongrass

PRECAUTIONS

Avoid use with children 6 years or younger; Avoid contact with mucous membranes; May cause skin irritation

MEDICINAL PROPERTIES

analgesic, antibacterial, antifungal, antiseptic, febrifuge, insecticidal, stimulant

IDEAL FOR TREATING

cold, fatigue, flu, foot odor, headache, insect infestations, oily skin

CLARY SAGE

Salvia sclarea

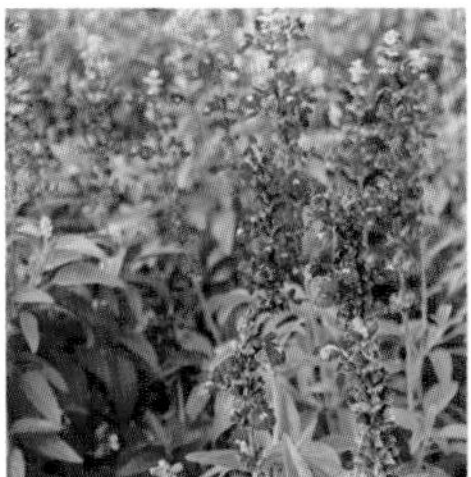

While clary sage costs a little more than some other popular essential oils, it's a must-have for female complaints such as PMS and hot flashes. Its ability to quiet and calm the mind makes it ideal for use when racing thoughts intrude. Its ability to regulate the skin's oil production makes it ideal for use in facial cleansers, natural dandruff remedies, and more.

BLENDS WELL WITH

bergamot, black pepper, geranium, juniper, lavender, lemon, pine

CAN BE SUBSTITUTED WITH

nutmeg, sage

PRECAUTIONS

Avoid use with children 6 years or younger; Avoid use if pregnant (other than when in labor); Avoid use if suffering from breast cancer; Avoid use before driving or operating machinery; Do not combine with alcohol

MEDICINAL PROPERTIES

antidepressant, antiseptic, bactericidal, digestive, emmenagogue, euphoric, hypotensive, sedative

IDEAL FOR TREATING

hot flashes, labor pains, menstrual cramps, PMS, sore throat, stress

CLOVE

Eugenia caryophyllata

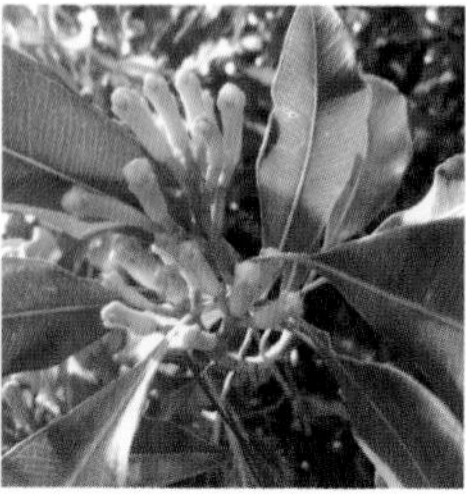

Just like the fragrant spice that makes a kitchen smell so good during holiday baking sessions, clove essential oil has a warm aroma that makes it a pleasure to use. Thanks to clove's strong antiseptic and disinfectant properties, it was an important tool for disease prevention centuries before modern medicines became available. Clove is my go-to for making natural dental-care products, and it makes a fantastic addition to an all-purpose cleaner.

BLENDS WELL WITH

basil, benzoin, cinnamon, clary sage, ginger, lavender, sandalwood

CAN BE SUBSTITUTED WITH

chamomile, cinnamon, juniper

PRECAUTIONS

Avoid use with children 6 years or younger; Avoid use if pregnant; May cause skin irritation

MEDICINAL PROPERTIES

analgesic, antiseptic, antispasmodic, disinfectant, insecticidal, stomachic

IDEAL FOR TREATING

bad breath, bronchitis, bruise, cold, diarrhea, flatulence, muscle aches, toothache

CYPRESS

Cupressus sempervirens

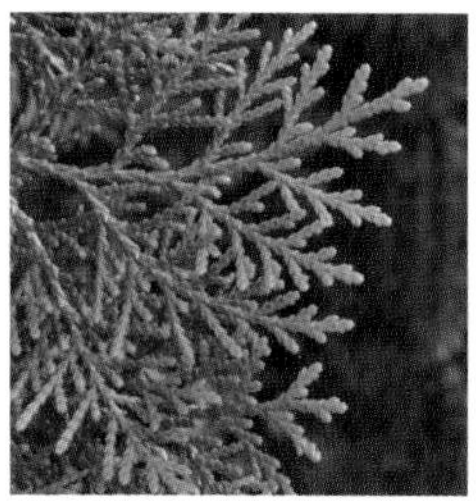

Cypress is a tall evergreen tree with dark green foliage. Cretans and Phoenicians used it extensively for homebuilding and boat building, Greeks favored it for carving statues of their gods, and Egyptians used it to make elegant sarcophagi. Cypress essential oil is extracted from the tree's needles and young twigs, which give it a fresh fragrance with just a hint of woody spice. It dispels angry moods when diffused, and its medicinal uses are many.

BLENDS WELL WITH

bergamot, clary sage, frankincense, juniper, rosemary

CAN BE SUBSTITUTED WITH

cedarwood, Roman chamomile

PRECAUTIONS

Avoid use if pregnant;
May cause skin irritation

MEDICINAL PROPERTIES

antiseptic, astringent, diuretic, emmenagogue, respiratory tonic, sedative, styptic, vasoconstrictor

IDEAL FOR TREATING

asthma, bronchitis, diarrhea, hemorrhoids, muscle cramps, nosebleed, oily skin, varicose veins, water retention, whooping cough

DAVANA

Artemisia pallens

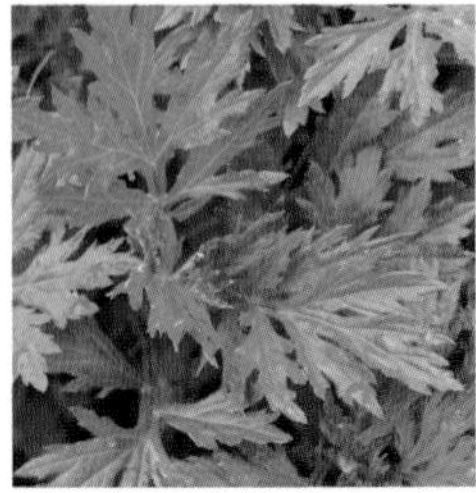

Davana is a fantastic essential oil known primarily for its unique fragrance, which smells different on each wearer. If you're interested in creating a signature fragrance for yourself, consider giving davana a try. When diffused, it takes on a sweet, slightly vanilla scent with hints of fruit and wood, plus an underlying camphorous note. When blended into perfumes, massage oils, and bath and body products, it promotes feelings of happiness and well-being.

BLENDS WELL WITH

bergamot, clove, cypress, ginger, lemon, mandarin, sweet orange

CAN BE SUBSTITUTED WITH

bergamot, vetiver

PRECAUTIONS

Avoid use if pregnant

MEDICINAL PROPERTIES

antidepressant, antiseptic, antiviral, disinfectant, emmenagogue, expectorant, relaxant, vulnerary

IDEAL FOR TREATING

anger, anxiety, cold, congestion, cough, cuts and scrapes, depression, flu, headache, PMS

DILL

Anethum graveolens, Anethum sowa

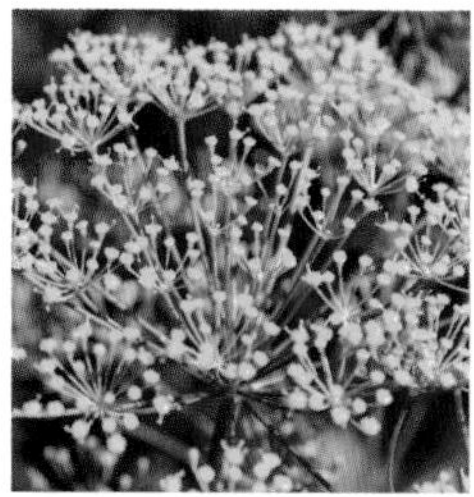

If you enjoy the flavor or fragrance of fresh dill, then you'll probably find this essential oil irresistible. Like the fresh herb, it's an excellent remedy for digestive upset, flatulence, and indigestion. Dill's sedative properties make it a good choice for dealing with nervousness and anxiety. It also has analgesic properties that make it ideal for soothing sore, stiff, or cramped muscles.

BLENDS WELL WITH

cinnamon, clove, lemon, lime, nutmeg, peppermint, spearmint, sweet orange

CAN BE SUBSTITUTED WITH

bergamot, ginger, spearmint

PRECAUTIONS

Generally considered safe

MEDICINAL PROPERTIES

antispasmodic, bactericidal, carminative, digestive, disinfectant, sedative

IDEAL FOR TREATING

colic, constipation, cramping, diarrhea, flatulence, hiccups, indigestion, insomnia, nervousness, tension headaches

EUCALYPTUS

Eucalyptus globulus

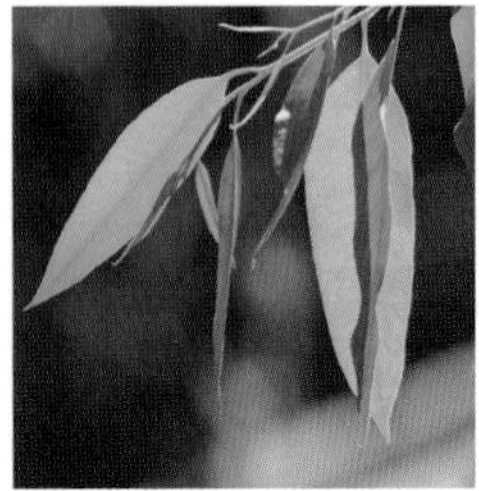

Made from the leaves and twigs of the eucalyptus tree, which is one of Australia's oldest native medicines, eucalyptus essential oil offers a multitude of uses. With its fresh, clean scent, it is a favorite for use as a natural deodorizer. A very popular ingredient in commercial vapor rubs and inhalants, eucalyptus also common in household cleaners and disinfectants.

BLENDS WELL WITH

chamomile, geranium, grapefruit, lavender, lemon

CAN BE SUBSTITUTED WITH

Eucalyptus radiata, lemon eucalyptus, tea tree

PRECAUTIONS

Avoid use with children 6 years or younger; Avoid use if pregnant or nursing; Avoid use if suffering from epilepsy or high blood pressure; Avoid use if suffering from an estrogen-dependent cancer

MEDICINAL PROPERTIES

analgesic, antibacterial, antiseptic, antiviral, decongestant, expectorant, febrifuge

IDEAL FOR TREATING

allergies, blisters, burns, chicken pox, cold, cuts and scrapes, flu, insect bites, muscle aches, skin infections

FIR NEEDLE

Abies balsamea, Abies alba

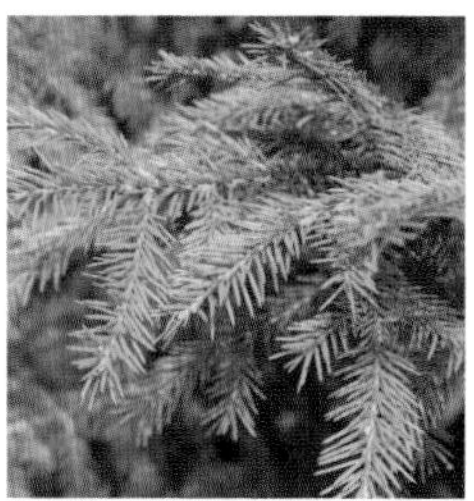

While fir needle offers a number of health benefits, it's one of my favorites mostly because of its beautiful, uplifting fragrance. Diffusing it—perhaps along with a drop of pine or cedarwood—gives your home a peaceful, enticing aroma. Like its close relative pine, fir needle is an excellent remedy for aches and pains. It's also a good choice for vapor therapy during cold and flu season.

BLENDS WELL WITH

benzoin, lavender, lemon, marjoram, pine, rosemary, sweet orange

CAN BE SUBSTITUTED WITH

cypress, juniper, pine

PRECAUTIONS

May cause skin irritation

MEDICINAL PROPERTIES

analgesic, antibacterial, antimicrobial, antiseptic, expectorant, stimulant

IDEAL FOR TREATING

body odor, bronchitis, cold, cough, flu, muscle soreness, muscle stiffness, sinusitis, sprain

FRANKINCENSE

Boswellia carteri

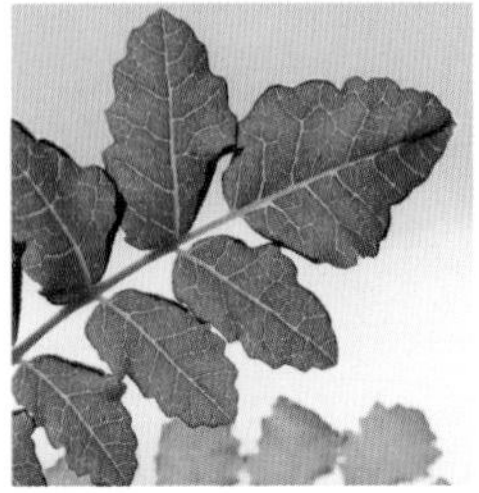

A pleasant, woody fragrance with spicy undertones makes frankincense an aromatherapy favorite. This essential oil is made from the resin of living frankincense trees, which also finds its way into incense. Diffuse it to promote a peaceful, meditative state of mind and to calm feelings of anxiety. Frankincense essential oil is fantastic for treating dry, cracked, or painful skin, and its ability to increase circulation makes it a top ingredient in healing salves.

BLENDS WELL WITH

benzoin, bergamot, ginger, lavender, lemon, myrrh, pine

CAN BE SUBSTITUTED WITH

helichrysum, myrrh, patchouli

PRECAUTIONS

Avoid use if pregnant

MEDICINAL PROPERTIES

antiseptic, astringent, carminative, digestive, diuretic, emmenagogue, expectorant, sedative

IDEAL FOR TREATING

anxiety, bronchitis, cold, cough, inflammation, minor wounds, night terrors, oily skin, stress

GERANIUM

Pelargonium odoratissimum

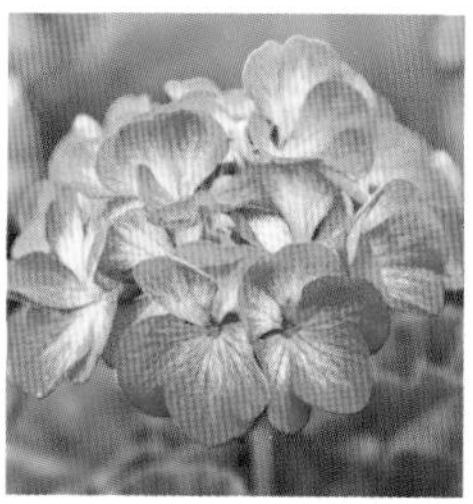

This fresh-smelling essential oil stimulates the adrenal cortex, helping balance turbulent emotions and focus a busy mind. Geranium also brings hormones into equilibrium and is helpful for treating PMS and menopause symptoms. Its ability to balance the skin's oil production makes it a favorite for skin care, and its vulnerary properties make it an excellent choice for healing minor cuts and sores. It's my go-to for treating bruises.

BLENDS WELL WITH

bergamot, cedarwood, clary sage, grapefruit, juniper, lemon, rosemary

CAN BE SUBSTITUTED WITH

rose geranium

PRECAUTIONS

Avoid use with children 6 years or younger; Not recommended for use during pregnancy; May cause skin irritation

MEDICINAL PROPERTIES

astringent, cicatrisant, diuretic, styptic, tonic, vermifuge, vulnerary

IDEAL FOR TREATING

acne, breast tenderness, bruises, burns, cellulite, eczema, menopause symptoms, PMS, postpartum depression, shingles

GINGER

Zingiberaceae officinale

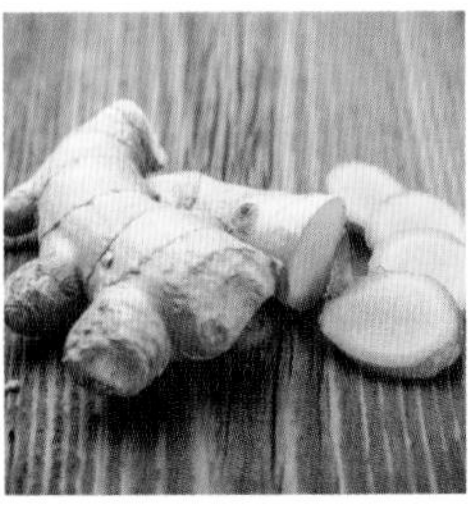

Muscle pain and stiffness are no match for ginger essential oil. Sourced from the same roots as those used to make powdered and candied ginger for cooking and baking, it offers a warm, spicy aroma that most people appreciate. Like the herb it comes from, ginger essential oil is an excellent treatment for nausea, making it a must-have for anyone who suffers from travel sickness.

BLENDS WELL WITH

bergamot, frankincense, lemon, orange, ylang-ylang

CAN BE SUBSTITUTED WITH

cardamom, peppermint, wild orange

PRECAUTIONS

Avoid sunlight after use; May cause skin irritation; Not recommended for use during pregnancy

MEDICINAL PROPERTIES

analgesic, anti-emetic, antiseptic, expectorant, febrifuge, laxative, tonic

IDEAL FOR TREATING

bruising, cold, colic, cramps, flu, hangover, indigestion, mild depression, nausea, sinusitis

GRAPEFRUIT

Citrus paradisi

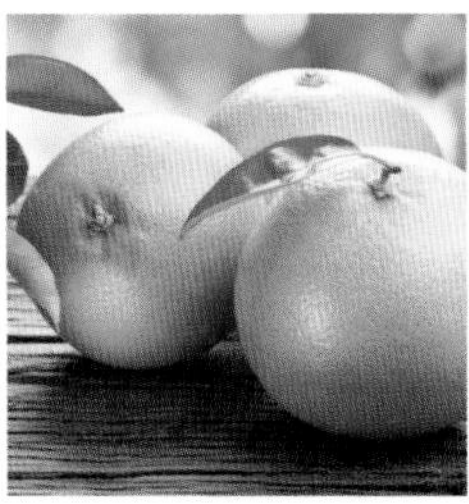

Just like the fruit it comes from, grapefruit essential oil offers a stimulating aroma that can improve a gloomy mood quickly. Because it contains plenty of vitamin C, grapefruit essential oil can contribute to a healthy immune system. Its diuretic property makes it useful for treating swollen feet and ankles and for clearing toxins from the body. Diffuse a few drops to deal with a headache or a hangover.

BLENDS WELL WITH

bergamot, frankincense, geranium, ginger, lavender, lemon, mandarin

CAN BE SUBSTITUTED WITH

bergamot, lemon, mandarin

PRECAUTIONS

Avoid sunlight after use; May cause skin irritation

MEDICINAL PROPERTIES

antidepressant, anti-infectious, antiseptic, aperitif, diuretic, lymphatic stimulant, tonic

IDEAL FOR TREATING

acne, cellulite, cold, cough, headache, jet lag, mild depression, moodiness, oily skin

HELICHRYSUM

Helichrysum angustifolium

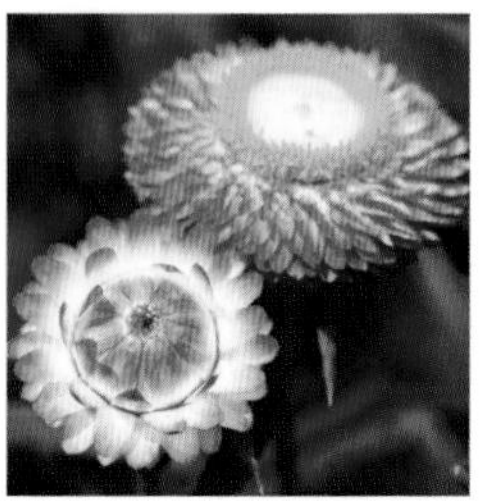

Sometimes referred to as immortelle or everlasting oil, helichrysum comes from an evergreen herb with a strong honey fragrance. Because it is highly aromatic, this plant was a favorite medieval strewing herb. Helichrysum essential oil eases minor strains and sprains, helps wounds heal quickly, fades scars, and makes an excellent addition to antiaging remedies. Diffuse a few drops to improve mental focus.

BLENDS WELL WITH
bergamot, clary sage, lavender, mandarin, Roman chamomile, rosewood

CAN BE SUBSTITUTED WITH
cypress, frankincense, myrrh

PRECAUTIONS
Generally considered safe

MEDICINAL PROPERTIES
analgesic, anti-allergenic, anti-inflammatory, astringent, cholagogue, diuretic, expectorant

IDEAL FOR TREATING
allergies, anxiety, asthma, boils, cough, eczema, fever, insect bites, minor wounds, sunburn

JASMINE

Jasminum grandiflorum

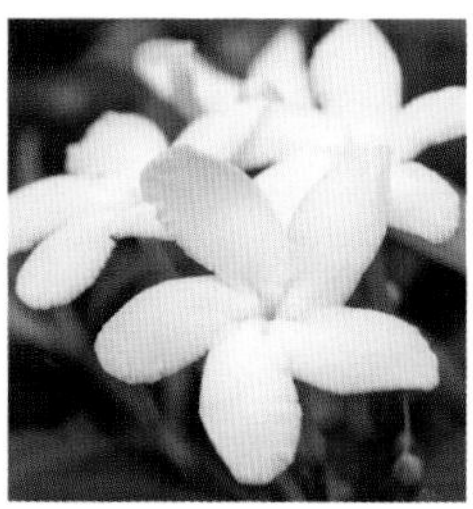

Jasmine is a powerful emmenagogue that shouldn't be used during pregnancy, but it proves indispensable during and after labor. Some doulas use jasmine to help encourage contractions and ease labor pains. It helps stimulate lactation, and if you suffer from postnatal depression, it is one of the best to have on hand. Jasmine essential oil is pricey, especially if you go for absolute instead of a blend; however, a little goes a long way.

BLENDS WELL WITH

bergamot, clary sage, cypress, frankincense, lemon, mandarin, sweet orange

CAN BE SUBSTITUTED WITH

clary sage, helichrysum, nutmeg

PRECAUTIONS

Avoid use if pregnant; Avoid use before driving or operating machinery; May cause headaches when used heavily

MEDICINAL PROPERTIES

antidepressant, antispasmodic, aphrodisiac, cicatrisant, emmenagogue, expectorant, parturient, sedative

IDEAL FOR TREATING

cold, cough, depression, enlarged prostate, flu, impotence, PMS, scars and stretch marks

JUNIPER

Juniperus communis

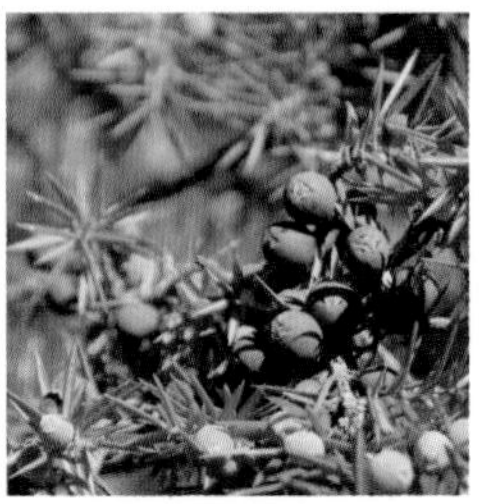

You may have seen junipers growing in your community. These fragrant evergreen shrubs are good for more than just landscaping, though. Their purple berries give gin its flavor, and they are commonly used in herbal medicine worldwide. Juniper essential oil can help improve acne, balance oily skin, and bring relief from other tough skin conditions, including psoriasis and eczema. It is among my favorite oils for soothing sore, overworked muscles.

BLENDS WELL WITH

cedarwood, clary sage, cypress, geranium, lavender

CAN BE SUBSTITUTED WITH

fir needle, pine, spruce

PRECAUTIONS

Avoid use with children 6 years or younger; Not recommended for use during pregnancy; Avoid use if suffering from kidney or liver disease

MEDICINAL PROPERTIES

antiseptic, astringent, bactericidal, diuretic, rubefacient, sudorific, vulnerary

IDEAL FOR TREATING

acne, back pain, bloating, dandruff, eczema, muscle spasms, oily skin, PMS, psoriasis, water retention

LAVENDER

Lavandula angustifolia

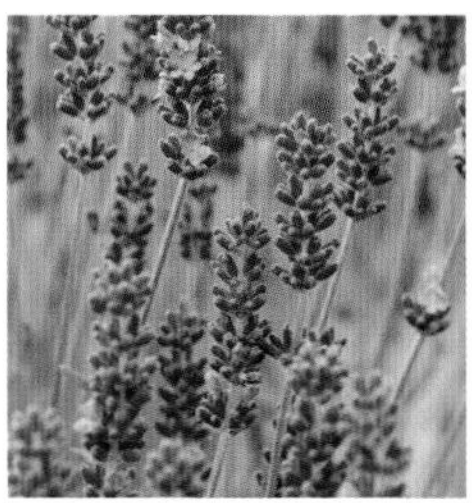

Perhaps best known for its ability to promote relaxation, lavender essential oil has a fresh, faintly floral aroma with strong herbal overtones and just a hint of camphor. This versatile essential oil is typically steam distilled from the leaves, flowers, and buds of the plant. It is one of the safest essential oils available and is suitable for use by every member of the family.

BLENDS WELL WITH

chamomile, eucalyptus, peppermint, rosemary, tea tree

CAN BE SUBSTITUTED WITH

hyssop, lavandin, spike lavender

PRECAUTIONS

Discontinue use if allergic reaction develops; Avoid use if suffering from an estrogen-dependent cancer; Avoid use before driving or operating machinery

MEDICINAL PROPERTIES

analgesic, antiseptic, antiviral, bactericidal, decongestant, hypotensive, sedative

IDEAL FOR TREATING

abscesses, acne, burns, cold, congestion, headaches, insect bites, insomnia, psoriasis, sunburn

LEMON

Citrus limonum

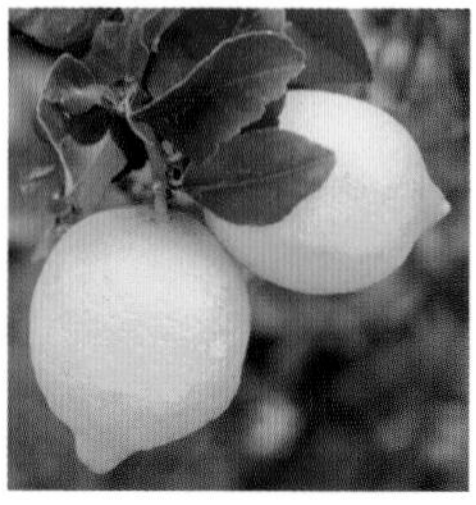

Offering a fresh, clean aroma that can send a bad mood packing, lemon essential oil is a favorite for aromatherapy and household use. Its ability to soothe tough headaches makes it a must-have, and its ability to ease cold and flu symptoms adds to its usefulness. Acne and oily skin are no match for its astringent property, and its ability to impart shine makes it a favored addition to hair products.

BLENDS WELL WITH

eucalyptus, fennel, geranium, juniper, lavender, orange, ylang-ylang

CAN BE SUBSTITUTED WITH

bergamot, grapefruit, lemongrass, mandarin

PRECAUTIONS

Avoid sunlight after use; May cause skin irritation

MEDICINAL PROPERTIES

anti-emetic, antimicrobial, antiseptic, bactericidal, diuretic, febrifuge, hypotensive

IDEAL FOR TREATING

asthma, cold, cold sores, cough, flu, headache, high blood pressure, indigestion, insect bites, migraine

LEMONGRASS

Cymbopogon citratus, Cymbopogon flexuosus

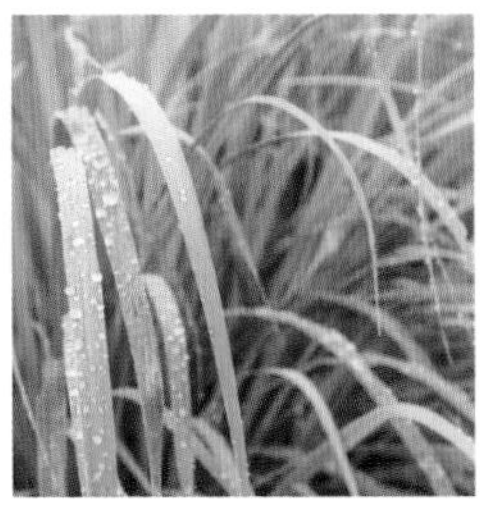

As a culinary herb, lemongrass imparts an intriguing flavor to a variety of foods. Essential oil made from this perennial grass is equally versatile, benefiting troubled skin, soothing sore muscles, and making quick work of jet lag, lethargy, and fatigue. Since it shares a bug-repelling chemical with citronella, lemongrass essential oil is an indispensable addition to homemade insect repellent recipes.

BLENDS WELL WITH

basil, cedarwood, geranium, ginger, lavender, tea tree, thyme

CAN BE SUBSTITUTED WITH

bergamot, grapefruit, lemon

PRECAUTIONS

Avoid use with children 6 years or younger; Avoid use if suffering from an estrogen-dependent cancer; May cause skin irritation

MEDICINAL PROPERTIES

analgesic, antidepressant, antimicrobial, antiseptic, bactericidal, fungicidal, insecticidal

IDEAL FOR TREATING

acne, athlete's foot, fatigue, fever, indigestion, laryngitis, muscle pain, nervous tension, ringworm, sore throat

LIME

Citrus aurantifolia

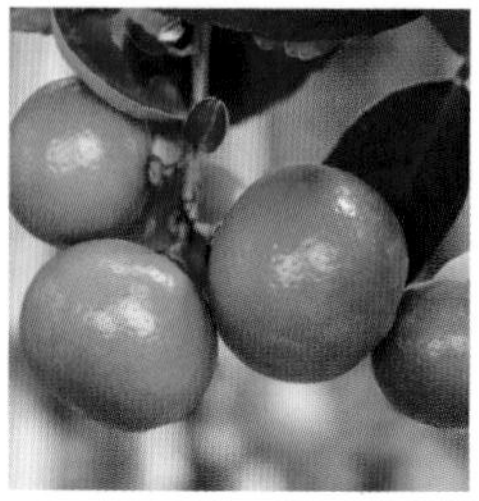

Just like the fruit, lime essential oil offers an enticing citrus aroma that most people enjoy. Like its close relatives lemon and mandarin, it has the ability to improve a sour mood. Try it for treating acne, insect bites, or spider veins, and use it with a hot compress if your muscles are feeling stiff and sore after a long day.

BLENDS WELL WITH
citronella, clary sage, lavender, lemon, nutmeg, rosemary, ylang-ylang

CAN BE SUBSTITUTED WITH
grapefruit, lemon, sweet orange

PRECAUTIONS
Avoid sunlight after use

MEDICINAL PROPERTIES
antibacterial, antidepressant, antiseptic, antiviral, disinfectant, febrifuge, tonic

IDEAL FOR TREATING
acne, bronchitis, cold, cold sores, cough, cut, exhaustion, muscle pain, oily skin, sinusitis

MANDARIN

Citrus reticulata

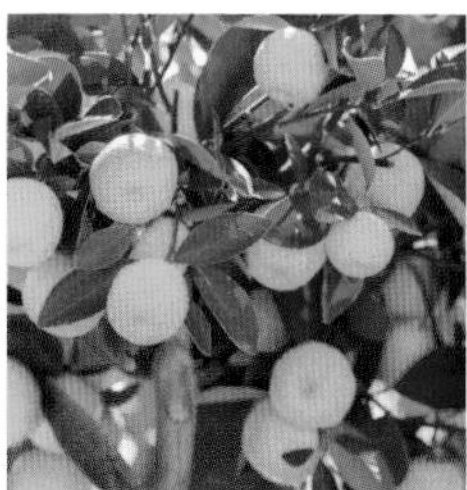

If you have young children, consider making mandarin essential oil one of the first oils you bring home. With its bright, fruity fragrance, it makes your home a cheery place to be. A parent's go-to for putting a quick stop to temper tantrums, it simultaneously soothes frazzled nerves. Besides improving everyone's mental state, it helps with digestive problems, including flatulence, constipation, and diarrhea. Diffuse it with lavender to send fussy children off to sleep.

BLENDS WELL WITH

bergamot, cinnamon, clary sage, frankincense, grapefruit, lavender, lemon

CAN BE SUBSTITUTED WITH

grapefruit, lemon, sweet orange

PRECAUTIONS

Avoid sunlight after use

MEDICINAL PROPERTIES

antimicrobial, antiseptic, antispasmodic, depurative, sedative, stomachic, tonic

IDEAL FOR TREATING

acne, cold, cough, flu, indigestion, nervousness, stress, stretch marks, temper tantrums, water retention

MARJORAM

Origanum majorana, Origanum hortensis

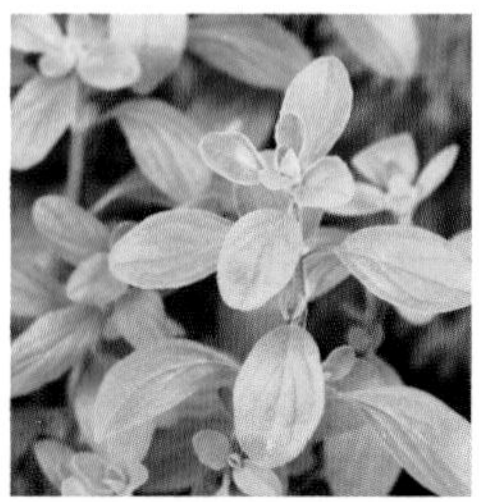

If marjoram sounds familiar to you, it's probably because you've used this herb in recipes. Like the savory leaves used for cooking, marjoram essential oil comes from a short, bushy Mediterranean herb. It is particularly useful for asthma, as it helps open the airways while promoting a sense of calm. Since marjoram essential oil is a natural muscle relaxant, it is excellent for back pain, menstrual cramps, and more.

BLENDS WELL WITH

bergamot, cedarwood, cypress, lavender, Roman chamomile

CAN BE SUBSTITUTED WITH

lemongrass, oregano, rosemary

PRECAUTIONS

Avoid use if pregnant; Avoid use before driving or operating machinery

MEDICINAL PROPERTIES

analgesic, antiseptic, antiviral, bactericidal, emmenagogue, expectorant, sedative, vasodilator

IDEAL FOR TREATING

asthma, bronchitis, congestion, cramps, headache, heartburn, insomnia, migraine, muscle spasms, sinusitis

MELISSA

Melissa officinalis

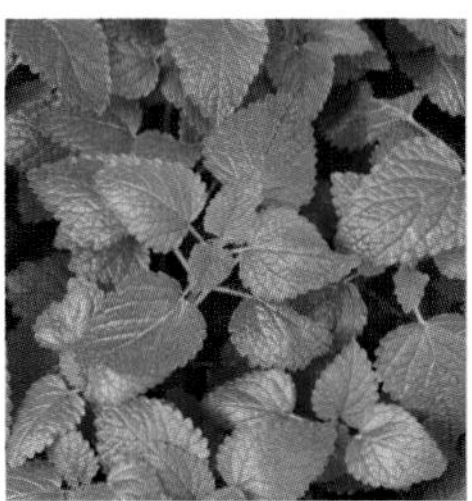

Also known as lemon balm and sometimes called sweet balm, melissa is a member of the mint family and shares some characteristics with peppermint and spearmint essential oils. As a powerful antibacterial agent, it is one of my go-to oils for whipping up natural household cleaners. It's also effective for pain relief and indigestion, and it possesses a mild sedative property that makes it useful for dealing with stress.

BLENDS WELL WITH

bergamot, frankincense, geranium, lemon, Roman chamomile, rose

CAN BE SUBSTITUTED WITH

catnip, peppermint, spearmint

PRECAUTIONS

Avoid use if pregnant; Avoid use before driving or operating machinery; May cause skin irritation

MEDICINAL PROPERTIES

analgesic, antifungal, antihistamine, antiseptic, antiviral, emmenagogue, sedative

IDEAL FOR TREATING

cold sores, depression, fever, flatulence, headache, herpes, indigestion, nausea, ringworm, stress

MYRRH

Commiphora myrrha, Commiphora molmol

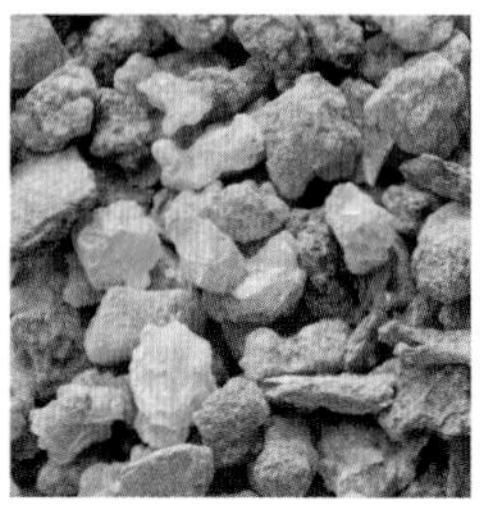

Although its exotic fragrance makes it a favorite in perfumery, myrrh is best enjoyed for its ability to soothe an array of physical and emotional ills. Its ability to stop bleeding is legendary; Greek soldiers took myrrh oil into battle, using it to treat wounds quickly. Painful skin conditions, athlete's foot, and gingivitis are just a few of the things myrrh is good for. Diffused in a sickroom, it makes cold symptoms more tolerable.

BLENDS WELL WITH

benzoin, clove, frankincense, lavender, sandalwood

CAN BE SUBSTITUTED WITH

frankincense, helichrysum, patchouli

PRECAUTIONS

Avoid use if pregnant

MEDICINAL PROPERTIES

anti-catarrhal, anti-inflammatory, antimicrobial, antiseptic, carminative, emmenagogue, expectorant, sedative

IDEAL FOR TREATING

abscesses, bronchitis, chapped skin, cold, cough, diaper rash, eczema, gingivitis, hemorrhoids, painful periods

NIAOULI

Melaleuca viridiflora, Melaleuca quinquenervia

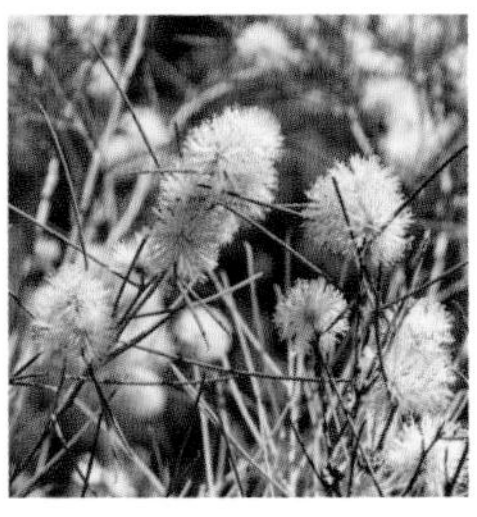

Niaouli essential oil comes from an Australian evergreen tree that looks and smells similar to eucalyptus. Its aroma is wonderfully uplifting, and its ability to clear congested nasal passages makes it nice to have on hand during cold and flu season. It helps with chest congestion, bronchitis, laryngitis, whooping cough, and even pneumonia symptoms. Its disinfectant property makes it ideal for use in first-aid salves.

BLENDS WELL WITH

fennel, juniper, lavender, peppermint, pine

CAN BE SUBSTITUTED WITH

eucalyptus, lemon eucalyptus, tea tree

PRECAUTIONS

Generally considered safe

MEDICINAL PROPERTIES

analgesic, antiseptic, bactericidal, decongestant, expectorant, febrifuge, vulnerary

IDEAL FOR TREATING

acne, asthma, bronchitis, burns, cold, cough, cuts and scrapes, insect bites, sinusitis, urinary tract infection

NUTMEG

Myristica fragrans

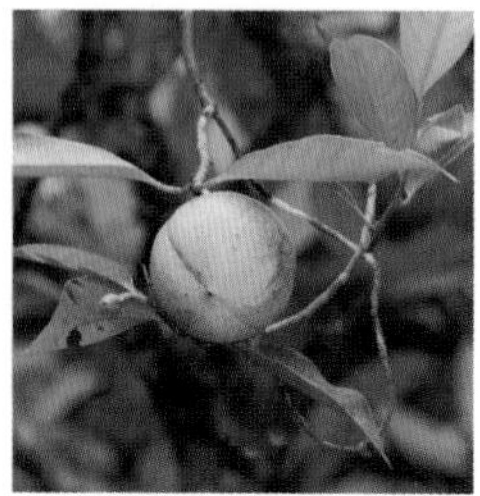

Nutmeg is a wonderful addition to any kitchen, and the essential oil that comes from this rich spice makes an equally outstanding addition to your aromatherapy arsenal. Its fragrance is purely delightful, with the ability to stimulate the mind, and its warming quality makes it a good choice for dealing with aches and pains. It is particularly useful when paired with a hot compress. Although it shouldn't be used while pregnant, like jasmine, nutmeg can be used to strengthen contractions during labor.

BLENDS WELL WITH

clary sage, clove, geranium, ginger, lime, mandarin, sweet orange

CAN BE SUBSTITUTED WITH

cinnamon bark, clove, ginger, jasmine

PRECAUTIONS

Avoid use if pregnant

MEDICINAL PROPERTIES

analgesic, antiseptic, antispasmodic, aphrodisiac, digestive, emmenagogue, laxative, parturient, stimulant

IDEAL FOR TREATING

constipation, diarrhea, flatulence, impotence, muscle soreness, muscle stiffness, oily hair, sprain, vomiting

OREGANO

Origanum vulgare

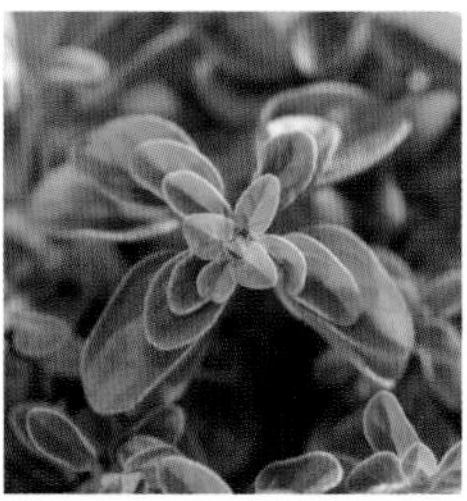

As a culinary herb, oregano imparts a delicious savory flavor. Despite its humble origins, it is one of the most powerful healing oils around, with antibacterial, antiviral, and immune-boosting properties that make it one of the best for dealing with infections. Blended into salves, it offers quick pain relief, and diffused or vaporized, it soothes cold and flu symptoms.

BLENDS WELL WITH

basil, cedarwood, citronella, cypress, lemongrass, Roman chamomile, rosemary

CAN BE SUBSTITUTED WITH

eucalyptus, tea tree, thyme

PRECAUTIONS

Avoid use if pregnant; Dilute well before use; May cause skin irritation

MEDICINAL PROPERTIES

analgesic, antibacterial, antifungal, antimicrobial, antiseptic, diuretic, emmenagogue, expectorant

IDEAL FOR TREATING

athlete's foot, bronchitis, cold, cough, flu, pneumonia, ringworm, strep throat, water retention, yeast infection

PATCHOULI

Pogostemon cablin

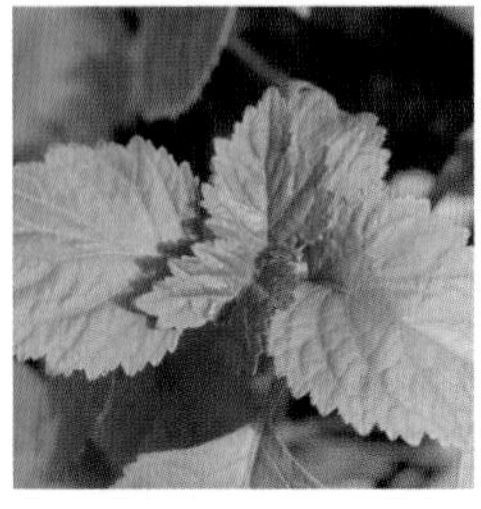

Patchouli is fantastic for imparting its warm, complex fragrance to bath and body products, but that's just the tip of the iceberg. Its antifungal properties make it an excellent treatment for athlete's foot, jock itch, and ringworm, and its decongestant properties make it a good oil for diffusing during cold and flu season. Patchouli also happens to be one of the best natural insect repellents there is, making it ideal for use in homemade bug sprays.

BLENDS WELL WITH

bergamot, cedarwood, geranium, jasmine, lemongrass, valerian, vetiver

CAN BE SUBSTITUTED WITH

citronella, eucalyptus, tea tree

PRECAUTIONS

Generally considered safe

MEDICINAL PROPERTIES

antibacterial, antifungal, anti-inflammatory, antiviral, febrifuge, insect repellant, laxative

IDEAL FOR TREATING

acne, athlete's foot, cellulite, congestion, constipation, eczema, fever, inflammation, insect bites, scars and stretch marks

PEPPERMINT

Mentha piperita

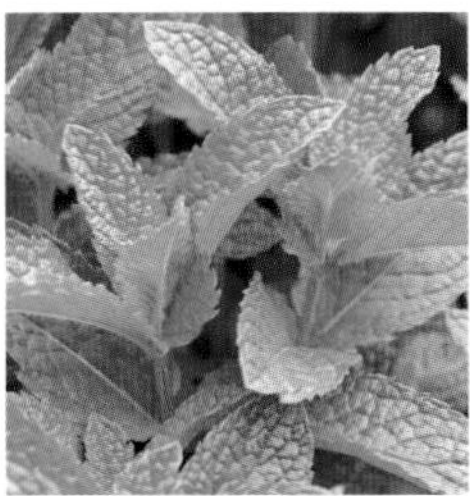

Cool, refreshing peppermint essential oil has a sharp, fresh fragrance with strong menthol overtones. A very inexpensive essential oil found in products ranging from toothpaste to candy, it also offers a variety of benefits to body and mind. Like the herb it's derived from, peppermint's ability to soothe the digestive system is well known, and its pleasant aroma makes it a pleasure to use. Just a whiff brings on a sense of mental alertness.

BLENDS WELL WITH

benzoin, eucalyptus, lavender, lemon, rosemary

CAN BE SUBSTITUTED WITH

cornmint, lemon balm, spearmint

PRECAUTIONS

Avoid use with children 6 years or younger; Avoid use if pregnant; Avoid use if suffering from epilepsy; May cause skin irritation; Avoid use with homeopathic remedies

MEDICINAL PROPERTIES

analgesic, antiseptic, astringent, digestive, emmenagogue, febrifuge, stimulant, vasoconstrictor

IDEAL FOR TREATING

asthma, bronchitis, cold, cramps, headache, migraine, muscle pain, nausea, skin irritation, sunburn

PINE

Pinus sylvestris

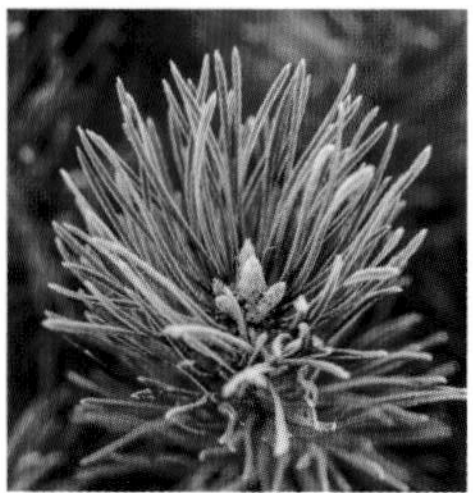

With a fresh, invigorating aroma, pine essential oil comes from the twigs and buds of a fragrant evergreen tree. Pine is such a powerful antiseptic and antimicrobial agent that it is used in commercial cleaning products, and it makes an excellent addition to homemade cleaning solutions you can use around the house. Pine isn't just for surfaces, though; it is an excellent choice for dealing with aches and pains, and it makes breathing easier in cases of asthma, bronchitis, cold, and cough.

BLENDS WELL WITH
cedarwood, eucalyptus, lavender, niaouli, rosemary

CAN BE SUBSTITUTED WITH
niaouli, Roman chamomile, tea tree

PRECAUTIONS
Avoid use with children 6 years and younger; Not recommended for use during pregnancy; May cause skin irritation

MEDICINAL PROPERTIES
antimicrobial, antiseptic, antiviral, bactericidal, disinfectant, diuretic, expectorant

IDEAL FOR TREATING
asthma, bronchitis, cold, cough, flu, laryngitis, minor sprains and strains, muscle aches, sinusitis, tendinitis

ROMAN CHAMOMILE

Anthemis nobilis

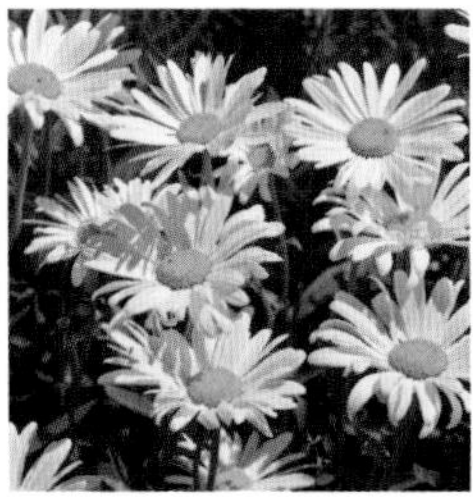

If you have ever enjoyed a cup of chamomile tea, then you have some familiarity with Roman chamomile's ability to calm frayed nerves. Its clean, crisp aroma is pleasant, with lightly fruity notes. Roman chamomile is one of just a few essential oils that lend themselves (well diluted, of course) to use in natural remedies for babies. Its thin consistency makes blending easy, and its pale blue color distinguishes it from its sapphire-colored relative, German chamomile.

BLENDS WELL WITH

clary sage, eucalyptus, geranium, grapefruit, lavender, lemon, tea tree

CAN BE SUBSTITUTED WITH

German chamomile, lavandin, lavender

PRECAUTIONS

Avoid use if pregnant; Avoid use before driving or operating machinery; May cause skin irritation

MEDICINAL PROPERTIES

analgesic, antidepressant, antiseptic, antispasmodic, digestive, emmenagogue, febrifuge, sedative

IDEAL FOR TREATING

abscesses, allergies, boils, colic, earache, flatulence, headache, insomnia, nausea, stress

ROSE

Rosa damascena, Rosa x damascena

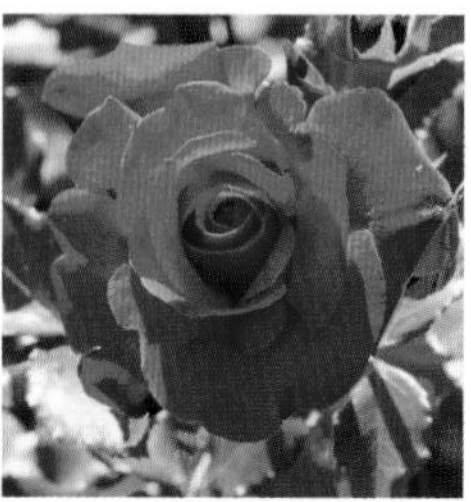

If you want to spoil yourself, go for rose absolute essential oil. Just one drop will add a soft, rose scent to creams and balms while helping heal problem skin. Rose is ideal for dry and aging facial skin. Diffuse it to fight depression, fear, and anger or to facilitate the grieving process after a loss. Blended rose oils aren't as powerful, but they do offer some of the same benefits. Check the Latin name before purchasing.

BLENDS WELL WITH
clove, davana, geranium, jasmine, mandarin

CAN BE SUBSTITUTED WITH
rose geranium, rose otto

PRECAUTIONS
Avoid use if pregnant

MEDICINAL PROPERTIES
antidepressant, antiseptic, antispasmodic, antiviral, aphrodisiac, emmenagogue, sedative, tonic

IDEAL FOR TREATING
allergies, broken capillaries, conjunctivitis, depression, dry skin, eczema, menopause, menstrual problems, migraine, nervous tension

ROSE GERANIUM

Pelargonium graveolens

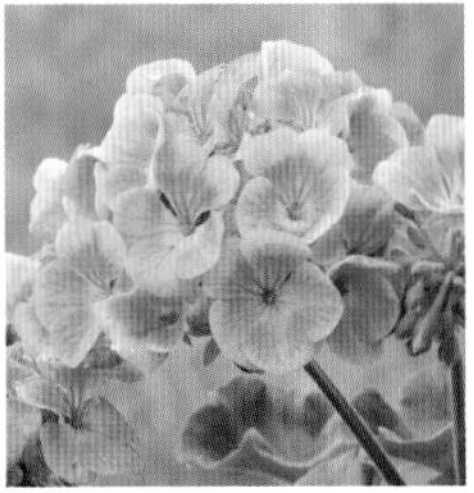

If you don't feel like springing for rose essential oil, give rose geranium a try. Its fragrance is purely delightful, and its ability to help compromised skin heal faster makes it useful for treating a variety of problems. Rose geranium is also a good stand-in for clary sage, offering some of the same hormone-balancing properties. Like its close relatives, this essential oil is a natural insect repellent.

BLENDS WELL WITH

basil, bergamot, carrot seed, cypress, rose, sweet orange, ylang-ylang

CAN BE SUBSTITUTED WITH

citronella, geranium

PRECAUTIONS

Avoid use if pregnant

MEDICINAL PROPERTIES

antidepressant, antifungal, antiseptic, astringent, diuretic, hormone balancing, insect repellent

IDEAL FOR TREATING

bruises, cellulite, cuts and scrapes, dry skin, eczema, hemorrhoids, lice, PMS, ringworm, water retention

ROSEMARY

Rosmarinus officinalis, Rosmarinus coronarium

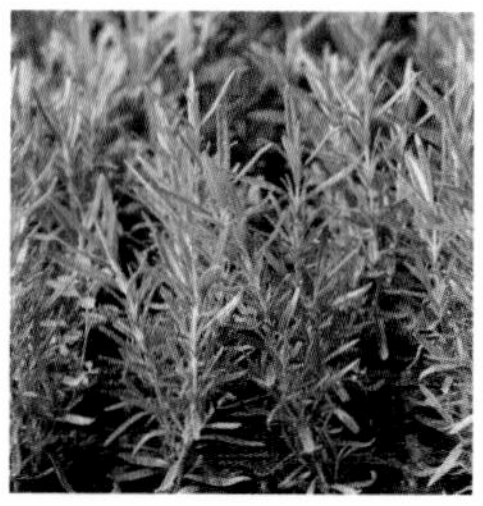

My go-to for getting through long work sessions while remaining mentally alert, rosemary essential oil also happens to be fantastic for treating a variety of physical ailments. Its ability to stimulate circulation makes it useful for easing headaches and stopping migraines. This same property makes it an excellent choice for dealing with spider veins and varicose veins. Rosemary essential oil eases breathing, too, making it fantastic for soothing asthma, bronchitis, and sinusitis symptoms.

BLENDS WELL WITH

cedarwood, geranium, lavender, lemongrass, peppermint

CAN BE SUBSTITUTED WITH

hyssop, peppermint, spearmint

PRECAUTIONS

Avoid use if pregnant; Avoid use if suffering from epilepsy; Avoid use if suffering from hypertension

MEDICINAL PROPERTIES

analgesic, antidepressant, astringent, cephalic, digestive, diuretic, emmenagogue, stimulant

IDEAL FOR TREATING

asthma, bronchitis, cold, cough, fatigue, headache, laryngitis, migraine, mild depression, sinus infection

SPEARMINT

Mentha spicata, Mentha viridis

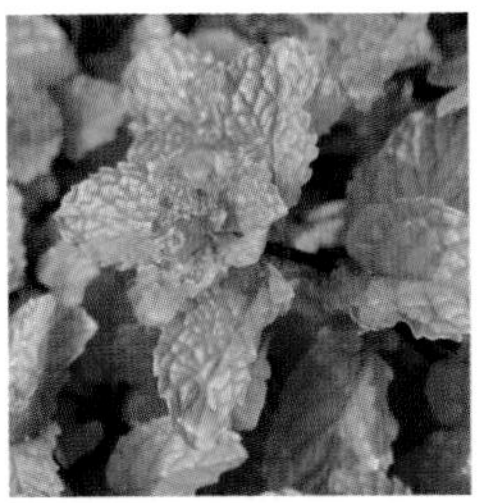

A sweeter, milder cousin of peppermint, spearmint is one of the best essential oils to keep on hand for children's complaints. Like peppermint, it stimulates the mind, and on skin it calms itchiness and helps heal dermatitis. Vomiting, diarrhea, colic, and flatulence can all be addressed by a bit of spearmint, and it's a good remedy for tension headaches and migraines. Spearmint is a mild muscle relaxant; try it for back spasms or hiccups.

BLENDS WELL WITH

basil, eucalyptus, lavender, lemon, rosemary

CAN BE SUBSTITUTED WITH

hyssop, melissa, peppermint

PRECAUTIONS

Avoid use if pregnant; Avoid use with homeopathic remedies

MEDICINAL PROPERTIES

antiseptic, antispasmodic, diuretic, emmenagogue, expectorant, febrifuge

IDEAL FOR TREATING

bronchitis, cold, colic, cough, diarrhea, fever, flu, headache, migraine, vomiting

SWEET ORANGE

Citrus sinensis

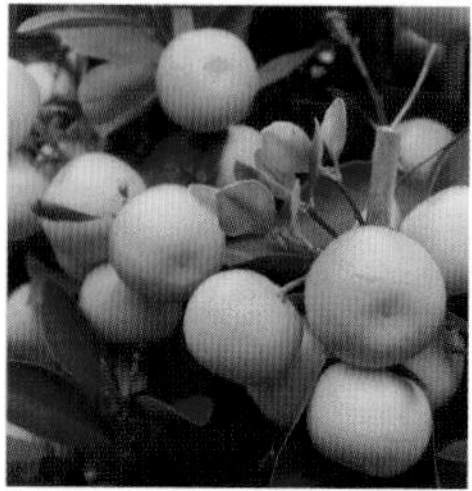

Not to be confused with bitter orange, wild orange, or neroli, sweet orange is a very inexpensive essential oil with a multitude of uses. In aromatherapy, it brings on feelings of happiness and security, and in the digestive tract, it calms indigestion, particularly the kind that accompanies stress. Sweet orange is a good cold and flu remedy that boosts the immune system, and like its cousin mandarin, it can help cranky children chill.

BLENDS WELL WITH

clove, frankincense, ginger, lemon, rosemary

CAN BE SUBSTITUTED WITH

grapefruit, mandarin, tangerine

PRECAUTIONS

Avoid sunlight after use

MEDICINAL PROPERTIES

antidepressant, anti-inflammatory, antiseptic, antispasmodic, diuretic, sedative, tonic

IDEAL FOR TREATING

acne, cold, dry skin, flu, indigestion, insomnia, skin irritation, stress, temper tantrums, water retention

TEA TREE

Melaleuca alternifolia

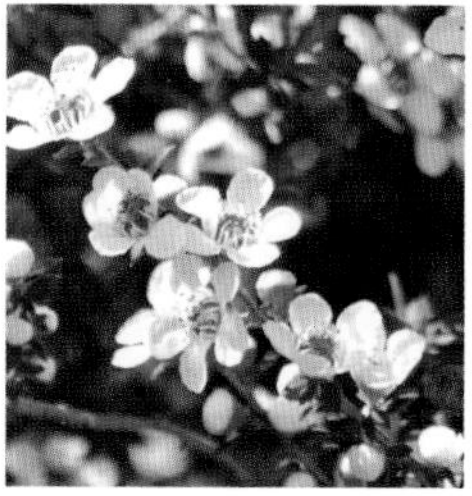

Widely known for its ability to improve compromised skin, tea tree essential oil is an excellent addition to a natural first-aid kit. An immune booster that also cleanses wounds, it fights bacteria, viruses, and fungi. Its pungent aroma gives way to a clean, spicy fragrance, making it a pleasure to use in natural household cleaners and bath products alike. If you must choose just a few essential oils, tea tree should be one of them.

BLENDS WELL WITH

clary sage, clove, geranium, lavender, rosemary

CAN BE SUBSTITUTED WITH

eucalyptus, lemon eucalyptus, manuka

PRECAUTIONS

Avoid use with children 2 years or younger; Avoid use if suffering from deep wounds; May cause skin irritation

MEDICINAL PROPERTIES

antifungal, antimicrobial, antiseptic, antiviral, bactericidal, expectorant, stimulant

IDEAL FOR TREATING

abscesses, acne, bronchitis, burns, cold, cold sores, flu, sinusitis, sunburn

THYME

Thymus vulgaris

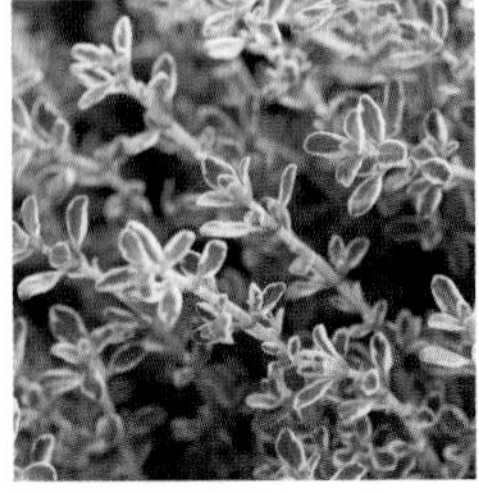

Its name derived from the Greek word thymos, *meaning perfume, thyme was used as incense in Grecian temples. Essential oil from this fragrant herb is highly potent, and when applied topically, it should be used in low concentrations. Its greatest value lies in treating upper respiratory and throat problems as well as lung issues; whooping cough, tonsillitis, and laryngitis can show improvement when thyme is part of your arsenal. Try it for night terrors, too.*

BLENDS WELL WITH

grapefruit, lavender, lemon, pine, rosemary

CAN BE SUBSTITUTED WITH

pine, Roman chamomile, tea tree

PRECAUTIONS

Avoid use if pregnant; May cause skin irritation

MEDICINAL PROPERTIES

antiseptic, bactericidal, carminative, cicatrisant, diuretic, emmenagogue, expectorant, tonic

IDEAL FOR TREATING

bronchitis, congestion, cough, flu, menstrual discomfort, mild depression, muscle aches, sinusitis, sore throat, tonsillitis

VALERIAN

Valeriana officinalis

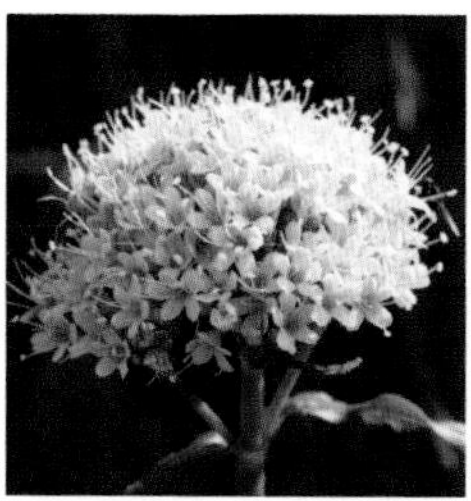

While valerian essential oil is best known for its usefulness as a natural sleep aid, it's also an outstanding tool for dealing with stress. Valerian can help balance turbulent emotions, making it helpful for dealing with the grouchiness that often accompanies PMS. Try it for teeth grinding, restlessness, and restless legs syndrome, too. Don't be put off by its pungent odor—the benefits are worth it.

BLENDS WELL WITH

cedarwood, fir needle, lavender, mandarin, patchouli, pine, rosemary

CAN BE SUBSTITUTED WITH

clary sage, ylang-ylang

PRECAUTIONS

Avoid use with children 6 years or younger; Avoid use if pregnant; Avoid use before driving or operating machinery

MEDICINAL PROPERTIES

antibacterial, antidepressant, diuretic, febrifuge, relaxant, sedative

IDEAL FOR TREATING

anger, anxiety, fever, headache, insomnia, muscle pain, PMS, restless legs syndrome, tendinitis, tension headache

VETIVER

Vetiveria zizanioides

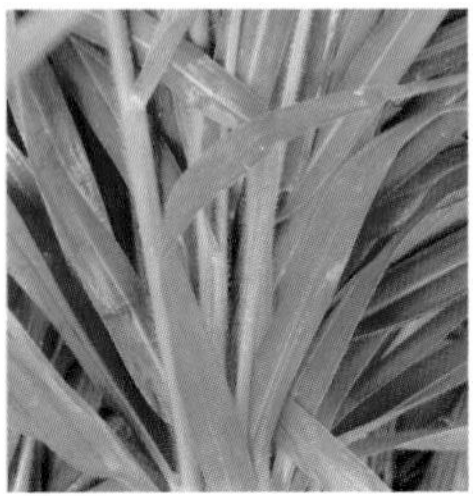

A very nice essential oil to keep on hand for stress and irritability, vetiver is also an excellent remedy for dealing with aches, pains, and insomnia. It balances and soothes dry, itchy skin and can help wounds heal faster. An excellent oil for new moms to keep on hand, vetiver helps ward off postpartum depression and can help you deal with the physical and emotional demands that come with caring for a newborn.

BLENDS WELL WITH

clary sage, grapefruit, lavender, mandarin, ylang-ylang

CAN BE SUBSTITUTED WITH

patchouli, rosewood, sandalwood

PRECAUTIONS

Avoid use before driving or operating machinery

MEDICINAL PROPERTIES

antiseptic, aphrodisiac, cicatrisant, nervine, sedative, tonic, vulnerary

IDEAL FOR TREATING

anger, anxiety, depression, dry skin, exhaustion, hyperactivity, insomnia, muscle pain, stress, tendinitis

YARROW

Achillea millefolium

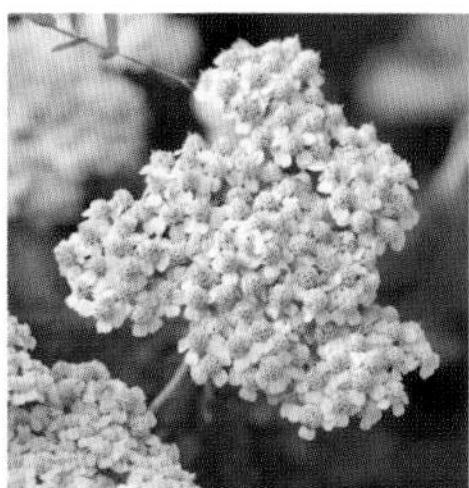

Yarrow has a clean, medicinal fragrance that you might find similar to commercial vapor rubs. This powerful essential oil is among the best for dealing with cold and flu symptoms. Try two or three drops in the diffuser or a vaporizer, or add it to a salve to use as a chest rub. If you suffer from spider veins, varicose veins, or hemorrhoids, yarrow can bring relief.

BLENDS WELL WITH

basil, cedarwood, eucalyptus, lavender, tea tree, thyme

CAN BE SUBSTITUTED WITH

eucalyptus, ginger, helichrysum

PRECAUTIONS

Not recommended for use during pregnancy; May cause skin irritation

MEDICINAL PROPERTIES

anti-inflammatory, antiseptic, antispasmodic, astringent, cicatrisant, digestive, expectorant, hypotensive

IDEAL FOR TREATING

acne, cold, cough, cuts and scrapes, cramps, indigestion, inflammation, insomnia, rashes, scars

YLANG-YLANG

Cananga odorata

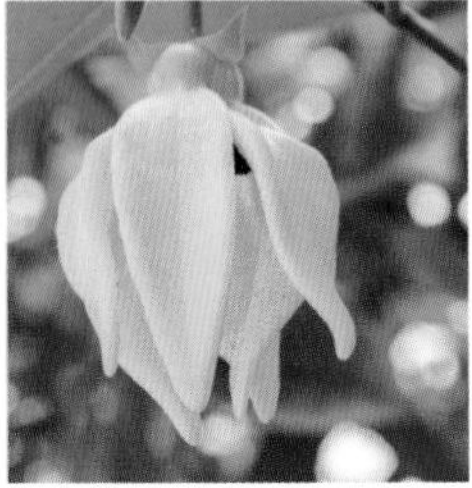

Treat yourself to a bottle of ylang-ylang essential oil, and you'll enjoy instant bliss. Offering a beautiful fragrance and lots of benefits for hair and skin, it also makes short work of mental and emotional strain. Ylang-ylang has a well-earned reputation as an aphrodisiac, so if you'd like to set the scene for romance, try diffusing a few drops in the bedroom.

BLENDS WELL WITH

bergamot, grapefruit, lavender, lemon, mandarin

CAN BE SUBSTITUTED WITH

jasmine, neroli, Roman chamomile

PRECAUTIONS

May cause headaches if overused; Avoid use before driving or operating machinery

MEDICINAL PROPERTIES

antibacterial, antidepressant, antiseptic, aphrodisiac, hypotensive, nervine, sedative

IDEAL FOR TREATING

anxiety, dandruff, dry skin, impotence, insomnia, itching, mild depression, oily skin and hair, stress, tension

GLOSSARY OF MEDICINAL PROPERTIES

ANALGESIC A substance that provides relief from pain, either by acting on the central nervous system or providing local numbing.

ANTI-ALLERGENIC A substance that will not aggravate allergies or that reduces their symptoms.

ANTI-ANXIETY A substance that can reduce feelings of anxiety.

ANTIBACTERIAL A substance that acts against bacteria by preventing or destroying them, or by slowing their multiplication.

ANTI-CATARRHAL A substance that helps remove excess mucus from the respiratory tract.

ANTIDEPRESSANT A substance that counteracts symptoms of mild depression.

ANTI-EMETIC A substance that reduces the severity or frequency of vomiting.

ANTIFUNGAL A substance that slows or prevents fungal growth. Also called fungicide.

ANTIHISTAMINE A substance that works by counteracting the body's natural reactions to allergens by opposing the activity of histamine receptors.

ANTI-INFECTIOUS A substance that provides protection against infections.

ANTI-INFLAMMATORY A substance that reduces inflammation.

ANTIMICROBIAL A substance that reduces microbial activity.

ANTISEBORRHEIC A substance that acts against dandruff and related skin conditions, providing relief from itching and improving the skin's appearance.

ANTISEPTIC A substance that acts against infections by slowing or stopping them.

ANTISPASMODIC A substance that helps stop cramping and muscle spasms.

ANTIVIRAL A substance that acts against viruses by preventing or destroying them, or by slowing their replication.

APERITIF A substance that stimulates the appetite.

APHRODISIAC A substance that can increase sexual desire or help improve the function of reproductive organs.

ASTRINGENT A substance that reduces inflammation and swelling by encouraging tissue to tighten or contract.

BACTERICIDE A substance that kills or destroys bacteria.

CALMATIVE A substance that can provide a calming effect.

CARMINATIVE A substance that reduces gas in the digestive tract, easing discomfort while reducing bloating and flatulence.

CEPHALIC A substance that can clear or stimulate the mind.

CHOLAGOGUE A substance that stimulates bile production.

CICATRISANT A substance that helps wounds heal quickly by promoting the rapid formation of scar tissue.

DECONGESTANT A substance that can relieve congestion.

DEPURATIVE A substance that facilitates waste removal by increasing lymph drainage and blood flow and supporting the liver and kidneys.

DETOXIFIER A substance that helps detoxify the body.

DIGESTIVE A substance that facilitates proper digestion by reducing inflammation or by stimulating or calming the digestive system.

DISINFECTANT A substance that destroys microorganisms on nonliving objects.

DIURETIC A substance that stimulates urine production, reducing bloating and swelling by removing excess water from the body.

EMMENAGOGUE A substance that increases circulation and prompts menstruation. Do not use emmenagogue essential oils during pregnancy.

EUPHORIC A substance that promotes a feeling of happiness.

EXPECTORANT A substance that stimulates a productive cough, helping expel phlegm and mucus from the lungs.

FEBRIFUGE A substance that physically reduces heat, lowering body temperature and helping prevent or reduce fevers.

HORMONE BALANCING A substance that promotes healthy hormonal balance.

HYPOTENSIVE A substance that reduces blood pressure. This property is sometimes referred to as hypotensor.

INSECT REPELLANT A substance that repels insects.

INSECTICIDAL A substance that kills insects.

LAXATIVE A substance that promotes bowel movements.

NERVINE A substance that therapeutically influences the nervous system, usually as a tonic or sedative that calms stress.

PARTURIENT A substance that can help with childbirth.

RELAXANT A substance that eases tension or promotes relaxation.

RESPIRATORY TONIC A substance that supports healthy breathing.

RUBEFACIENT A substance that dilates capillaries, increasing blood circulation and causing a warming sensation. Skin often reddens when rubefacients are applied.

SEDATIVE A substance that has a calming, soothing effect, or one that promotes deep relaxation or sleep.

STIMULANT A substance that offers an enlivening effect to the body and mind.

STOMACHIC A substance that helps improve appetite while aiding digestion.

STYPTIC A substance that stops external bleeding.

SUDORIFIC A substance capable of causing or increasing perspiration by stimulating the sweat glands.

TONIC A substance that tones the body in general or affects just one area; often has a stimulating, restorative effect.

VASOCONSTRICTOR A substance that eases inflammation by causing blood vessels within the application site to contract.

VASODILATOR A substance that relaxes muscles by causing blood vessels within the application site to widen.

VERMIFUGE A substance that expels intestinal worms.

VULNERARY A substance that helps heal sores, cuts, scrapes, and other open wounds.

AILMENTS AND OILS QUICK-REFERENCE GUIDE

AILMENT & SUGGESTED ESSENTIAL OILS	METHODS OF APPLICATION
ABSCESS	
Bergamot, cajuput, cedarwood, cypress, geranium, grapefruit, lavender, myrrh, Roman chamomile, tea tree	Bath, compress, direct application, massage
ACNE	
Benzoin, bergamot, cedarwood, clove, cypress, geranium, grapefruit, juniper, lavender, lemon, lemongrass, mandarin, niaouli, Roman chamomile, sweet orange, tea tree	Bath (body acne), direct application
ALLERGIES	
Anise, eucalyptus, helichrysum, peppermint, Roman chamomile, tea tree	Bath, inhalation, vaporization
ANXIETY	
Basil, bergamot, catnip, cedarwood, clary sage, frankincense, jasmine, lavender, orange, patchouli, rose	Bath, inhalation, massage, vaporization
ASTHMA	
Cajuput, cypress, frankincense, geranium, helichrysum, lavender, lemon, marjoram, niaouli, peppermint, pine, rosemary	Bath, inhalation, massage, vaporization
ATHLETE'S FOOT	
Clove, lavender, myrrh, oregano, patchouli, tea tree	Bath, direct application, massage, spray on

AILMENT & SUGGESTED ESSENTIAL OILS	METHODS OF APPLICATION
BACK PAIN	
Clary sage, clove, cypress, eucalyptus, ginger, juniper, lemongrass, peppermint, Roman chamomile, rosemary, spearmint, thyme, vetiver	Bath, compress, direct application
BAD BREATH	
Clove, lavender, lemon, orange, peppermint, spearmint	Gargle, spray
BEE STING	
Cajuput, clove, lavender, lemongrass, peppermint, Roman chamomile	Bath, direct application, spray on
BLACKHEADS	
Cajuput, clary sage, juniper, lavender, lemon, lemongrass, mandarin, sweet orange, tea tree	Compress, direct application
BLISTER	
Eucalyptus, helichrysum, lavender, myrrh, Roman chamomile	Bath, compress, direct application, spray on
BLOATING OR CRAMPING	
Clary sage, cypress, ginger, grapefruit, juniper, lavender, lemon, mandarin, marjoram, peppermint, pine, Roman chamomile	Bath, compress, direct application, massage
BODY ODOR	
Fir needle, lavender, peppermint, spearmint, tea tree, vetiver, ylang-ylang	Bath, direct application, massage, powder, spray on

AILMENT & SUGGESTED ESSENTIAL OILS	METHODS OF APPLICATION
BRONCHITIS	
Cajuput, cedarwood, clove, cypress, eucalyptus, frankincense, marjoram, myrrh, niaouli, peppermint, pine, rosemary, spearmint, tea tree, thyme	Bath, inhalation, massage, vaporization
BRUISE	
Clove, cypress, geranium, ginger, helichrysum, lavender, lemongrass, vetiver	Compress, direct application, massage, spray on
BURN	
Eucalyptus, frankincense, geranium, helichrysum, lavender, niaouli, tea tree	Compress, direct application, spray on
CHAPPED LIPS	
Frankincense, helichrysum, lavender, myrrh, Roman chamomile	Direct application
CHICKEN POX	
Bergamot, eucalyptus, lavender, Roman chamomile	Bath, compress, direct application
COLD	
Bergamot, cajuput, cedarwood, clove, eucalyptus, frankincense, ginger, grapefruit, lavender, lemon, mandarin, marjoram, myrrh, niaouli, peppermint, pine, rosemary, spearmint, sweet orange, tea tree, thyme	Bath, inhalation, massage, vaporization
COLD SORE	
Geranium, lavender, lemon, melissa, tea tree	Direct application

AILMENT & SUGGESTED ESSENTIAL OILS	METHODS OF APPLICATION
COLIC	
Dill, geranium, ginger, lavender, Roman chamomile, spearmint	Bath, direct application, massage
CONJUNCTIVITIS	
Clary sage, Roman chamomile	Compress, vaporization
CONSTIPATION	
Ginger, lemon, mandarin, peppermint, rosemary, spearmint, sweet orange	Bath, direct application, massage
COUGH	
Cajuput, cedarwood, eucalyptus, frankincense, ginger, grapefruit, helichrysum, lemon, mandarin, myrrh, niaouli, peppermint, pine, Roman chamomile, rosemary, spearmint, thyme	Bath, compress, direct application, vaporization
CRADLE CAP	
Lavender, myrrh	Direct application
CUT	
Eucalyptus, frankincense, helichrysum, lavender, niaouli, tea tree, thyme	Compress, direct application
DANDRUFF	
Cedarwood, juniper, lavender, lemon, myrrh, pine, rosemary, tea tree, thyme, ylang-ylang	Add to hair products, rinse, scalp massage
DIAPER RASH	
Frankincense, lavender, myrrh, Roman chamomile	Bath, compress, direct application

AILMENT & SUGGESTED ESSENTIAL OILS	METHODS OF APPLICATION
DIARRHEA	
Clove, cypress, eucalyptus, geranium, lavender, peppermint, Roman chamomile, spearmint	Bath, massage
DRY SKIN	
Frankincense, geranium, lavender, myrrh, sweet orange, vetiver, ylang-ylang	Bath, direct application, massage
EAR INFECTION	
Eucalyptus, lavender, rosemary, tea tree, thyme	Bath, compress, direct application, massage
EARACHE	
Lavender, Roman chamomile, tea tree, thyme	Compress, direct application, massage
ECZEMA	
Benzoin, bergamot, carrot seed, geranium, helichrysum, juniper, lavender, myrrh, peppermint, spearmint, sweet orange	Bath, direct application, massage
EXHAUSTION	
Frankincense, grapefruit, lavender, lemongrass, mandarin, myrrh, peppermint, rosemary, spearmint, sweet orange, vetiver, ylang-ylang	Bath, direct application, inhalation, massage, vaporization
FEVER	
Eucalyptus, ginger, helichrysum, lemon, lemongrass, patchouli, peppermint, spearmint	Compress, direct application, inhalation, vaporization

AILMENT & SUGGESTED ESSENTIAL OILS	METHODS OF APPLICATION
FLATULENCE	
Clove, ginger, nutmeg, peppermint, Roman chamomile, spearmint	Bath, direct application, massage
FLU	
Bergamot, cypress, eucalyptus, ginger, lavender, lemon, mandarin, peppermint, pine, spearmint, sweet orange, tea tree, thyme	Bath, direct application, inhalation, massage, vaporization
FROSTBITE	
Clove, geranium, lavender	Bath, direct application
HAND-FOOT-MOUTH DISEASE	
Cypress, lavender, Roman chamomile	Bath, direct application
HAY FEVER	
Eucalyptus, niaouli, peppermint, tea tree	Direct application, inhalation, vaporization
HEADACHE	
Cajuput, grapefruit, lavender, lemon, marjoram, peppermint, Roman chamomile, rosemary, spearmint	Bath, direct application, inhalation, massage, vaporization
HEARTBURN	
Ginger, marjoram, peppermint, spearmint	Direct application, massage
HEAT RASH	
Eucalyptus, lavender, Roman chamomile	Bath, direct application, spray on

AILMENT & SUGGESTED ESSENTIAL OILS	METHODS OF APPLICATION
HEMORRHOIDS	
Cypress, lavender, myrrh, tea tree	Bath, direct application
HICCUPS	
Dill, ginger, mandarin, peppermint, Roman chamomile, spearmint	Bath, inhalation, vaporization
HIVES	
Cypress, lavender, myrrh, Roman chamomile	Bath, direct application, massage
HOT FLASHES	
Clary sage, peppermint, spearmint	Direct application, inhalation, massage, vaporization
IMPETIGO	
Eucalyptus, lavender, myrrh, tea tree	Bath, direct application
INDIGESTION	
Basil, ginger, lemon, lemongrass, mandarin, peppermint, Roman chamomile, spearmint, sweet orange	Bath, direct application, inhalation, vaporization
INFLAMMATION	
Clove, frankincense, lavender, myrrh, patchouli, thyme	Bath, direct application, inhalation, massage, vaporization
INGROWN HAIR	
Lavender, Roman chamomile, tea tree	Bath, direct application, scrub

AILMENT & SUGGESTED ESSENTIAL OILS	METHODS OF APPLICATION
INGROWN TOENAIL	
Frankincense, lavender, myrrh, tea tree	Bath, direct application
INSECT BITES	
Eucalyptus, helichrysum, lavender, lemon, niaouli, peppermint, spearmint, tea tree	Bath, direct application, spray on
INSOMNIA	
Jasmine, lavender, marjoram, Roman chamomile, valerian, vetiver, yarrow, ylang-ylang	Bath, direct application, inhalation, vaporization
JET LAG	
Grapefruit, lavender, lemongrass, peppermint, Roman chamomile, spearmint, sweet orange, vetiver, ylang-ylang	Bath, direct application, inhalation, massage, vaporization
JOINT PAIN	
Clove, juniper, peppermint, pine, spearmint, vetiver	Bath, compress, direct application, massage
KERATOSIS PILARIS	
Clary sage, geranium, juniper, myrrh, rose, rose geranium	Bath, direct application, scrub
LARYNGITIS	
Eucalyptus, ginger, lemongrass, myrrh, peppermint, pine, rosemary, spearmint, tea tree, thyme	Bath, direct application, inhalation, massage, vaporization

AILMENT & SUGGESTED ESSENTIAL OILS	METHODS OF APPLICATION
LEG CRAMPS	
Cypress, juniper, lavender, marjoram, peppermint, pine	Bath, direct application, massage
LICE	
Geranium, lavender, rose geranium, thyme, tea tree	Direct application, mix with hair products
MENSTRUAL CRAMPS	
Clary sage, cypress, lavender, myrrh, peppermint, pine, spearmint, sweet orange	Bath, direct application, massage
MIGRAINE	
Lavender, lemon, marjoram, peppermint, rosemary, spearmint	Bath, direct application, inhalation, massage, vaporization
MORNING SICKNESS	
Lemongrass, spearmint	Bath, inhalation, vaporization
MOTION SICKNESS	
Ginger, peppermint, Roman chamomile, spearmint	Direct application, inhalation, vaporization
MUSCLE SORENESS	
Clary sage, clove, eucalyptus, ginger, juniper, lemongrass, peppermint, pine, spearmint, thyme, vetiver	Bath, compress, direct application, massage

AILMENT & SUGGESTED ESSENTIAL OILS	METHODS OF APPLICATION
MUSCLE SPASMS	
Clary sage, clove, cypress, juniper, lavender, marjoram, peppermint, pine, spearmint, sweet orange	Bath, compress, direct application, massage
MUSCLE STIFFNESS	
Clove, cypress, eucalyptus, lavender, lemongrass, peppermint, pine, spearmint, thyme, vetiver	Bath, compress, direct application, massage
NAIL FUNGUS	
Clove, lavender, lemongrass, oregano, tea tree	Bath, direct application
NAUSEA	
Anise, cajuput, ginger, peppermint, Roman chamomile, spearmint	Bath, direct application, inhalation, massage
NIGHT TERRORS	
Frankincense, lavender, mandarin, Roman chamomile, sweet orange, thyme	Bath, direct application, inhalation, massage, vaporization
NOSEBLEED	
Cypress, helichrysum, lavender	Compress, direct application
OILY SKIN	
Bergamot, cajuput, citronella, cypress, frankincense, grapefruit, juniper, lavender, lemon, lime, tea tree, ylang-ylang	Add to skin products, direct application

AILMENT & SUGGESTED ESSENTIAL OILS	METHODS OF APPLICATION
PNEUMONIA	
Frankincense, marjoram, myrrh, niaouli, peppermint, spearmint, tea tree	Bath, direct application, inhalation, massage, vaporization
POISON IVY/POISON OAK	
Lavender, peppermint, spearmint, tea tree	Bath, spray on
POSTPARTUM DEPRESSION	
Bergamot, cinnamon bark, davana, geranium, ginger, grapefruit, lavender, lemon, mandarin, Roman chamomile, rosemary, spearmint, sweet orange, vetiver, ylang-ylang	Bath, direct application, inhalation, massage, vaporization
PREMENSTRUAL SYNDROME (PMS)	
Basil, bergamot, clary sage, davana, geranium, grapefruit, jasmine, juniper, lavender, mandarin, sweet orange, vetiver, ylang-ylang	Bath, direct application, inhalation, massage, vaporization
PSORIASIS	
Bergamot, cajuput, cedarwood, juniper, lavender, myrrh, vetiver	Bath, direct application, massage
RAZOR BUMPS	
Helichrysum, lavender, myrrh, tea tree, yarrow	Bath, direct application, massage
RESTLESS LEGS SYNDROME	
Clary sage, frankincense, lavender, marjoram, Roman chamomile, valerian, ylang-ylang	Bath, direct application, massage

AILMENT & SUGGESTED ESSENTIAL OILS	METHODS OF APPLICATION
RINGWORM	
Lavender, lemongrass, melissa, myrrh, oregano, patchouli, rose geranium, tea tree, thyme	Bath, direct application, spray on
SHINGLES	
Clove, geranium, lavender, myrrh	Bath, direct application, spray on
SINUSITIS	
Cajuput, eucalyptus, fir needle, ginger, lime, myrrh, niaouli, peppermint, pine, rosemary, spearmint, tea tree, thyme	Bath, direct application, inhalation, vaporization
SORE THROAT	
Cajuput, clary sage, clove, lemon, lemongrass, peppermint, pine, spearmint	Bath, direct application, inhalation, vaporization
SPLINTER	
Cedarwood, frankincense, helichrysum, lavender, myrrh, Roman chamomile	Bath, direct application, inhalation, vaporization
SPRAIN	
Clove, fir needle, juniper, lavender, peppermint, pine, spearmint, thyme	Bath, compress, direct application, massage
STOMACHACHE	
Ginger, peppermint, Roman chamomile, spearmint, sweet orange, vetiver	Bath, compress, direct application, inhalation, massage, vaporization

AILMENT & SUGGESTED ESSENTIAL OILS	METHODS OF APPLICATION
STREP THROAT	
Eucalyptus, lavender, lemon, lemongrass, myrrh, oregano, peppermint, pine, spearmint, thyme	Bath, direct application, inhalation, vaporization
STRESS	
Bergamot, catnip, clary sage, frankincense, lavender, lemon, mandarin, niaouli, peppermint, Roman chamomile, rosemary, spearmint, sweet orange, vetiver, ylang-ylang	Bath, direct application, inhalation, massage, vaporization
STRETCH MARKS	
Geranium, helichrysum, jasmine, lavender, mandarin, myrrh, patchouli, rose, vetiver	Direct application, massage
STUFFY NOSE	
Eucalyptus, jasmine, lavender, lemon, marjoram, niaouli, peppermint, pine, rose, rosemary, spearmint	Bath, direct application, inhalation, vaporization
STY	
Lavender, myrrh, Roman chamomile	Compress, vaporization
SUNBURN	
Helichrysum, lavender, myrrh, peppermint, Roman chamomile, spearmint, tea tree	Direct application, spray on
SWIMMER'S EAR	
Eucalyptus, lavender, rosemary, thyme	Compress, massage

AILMENT & SUGGESTED ESSENTIAL OILS	METHODS OF APPLICATION
SWOLLEN ANKLES OR FEET	
Grapefruit, lemon, mandarin, pine, peppermint, spearmint, sweet orange, thyme	Bath, compress, direct application, massage, spray on
TEETH GRINDING	
Lavender, peppermint, Roman chamomile, spearmint, sweet orange, thyme, valerian, vetiver, ylang-ylang	Direct application, inhalation, massage, vaporization
TENDINITIS	
Helichrysum, juniper, lemongrass, peppermint, pine, spearmint, thyme, vetiver	Bath, compress, direct application, massage
THRUSH	
Lavender, lemon, Roman chamomile, thyme	Direct application, gargle, oil pulling
VOMITING	
Anise, ginger, nutmeg, peppermint, Roman chamomile, spearmint	Bath, direct application, inhalation, vaporization
WATER RETENTION	
Carrot seed, cypress, geranium, grapefruit, juniper, lemon, mandarin, pine, spearmint, sweet orange, thyme	Bath, direct application, massage
YEAST INFECTION	
Lavender, myrrh, tea tree	Bath, poultice

ESSENTIAL OILS BRANDS

There are many excellent essential oil brands available, but it can be difficult to determine which are widely trusted. To make that task easier, here are ten of the most popular.

Aura Cacia

DESCRIPTION Founded in 1982, Aura Cacia offers an extensive line of essential oils and products containing essential oils.

WHERE TO BUY You can purchase Aura Cacia products online and in select stores. Many brick-and-mortar retailers carry only a portion of the essential oils the company produces.

RATINGS AND REVIEWS Customers give Aura Cacia high marks for its reasonable prices and for the quality of the essential oils they produce.

dōTERRA

DESCRIPTION dōTERRA was founded in 2008, making it a relatively new company. dōTERRA offers numerous single oils as well as several signature blends and kits containing an array of the most popular oils and blends.

WHERE TO BUY You can purchase dōTERRA essential oils only from independent product consultants, either in person or online. Many dōTERRA consultants sell on Amazon, eBay, and similar sites.

RATINGS AND REVIEWS dōTERRA receives high marks for quality but lower marks for pricing. The company's kits receive excellent reviews.

OTHER Use caution when purchasing dōTERRA essential oils online. Some consumers have reported that they've received fake products from certain sellers, so check seller ratings before placing an order.

Edens Garden

DESCRIPTION Edens Garden offers a good selection of essential oil singles, synergistic blends, and carrier oils. Starter kits are also available.

WHERE TO BUY You can purchase Edens Garden essential oils online.

RATINGS AND REVIEWS Customers give this company high marks for quality, price, and service.

OTHER Use caution if purchasing Edens Garden products from anywhere other than their website or another official storefront such as Amazon. Products labeled as Edens Garden that are purchased from another seller may be adulterated or overpriced.

Heritage Essential Oils

DESCRIPTION Heritage Essential Oils is a small family-owned company that provides a good selection of single essential oils, blends, and products made with essential oils. Custom blends are available, as are organic essential oils and wild-crafted essential oils.

WHERE TO BUY You can purchase Heritage Essential Oils online.

RATINGS AND REVIEWS Customers give this company high marks for quality and value.

Mountain Rose Herbs

DESCRIPTION Mountain Rose Herbs has been offering certified organic products since 1987. An extensive selection of single essential oils are available along with blended oils and products containing them.

WHERE TO BUY You can purchase Mountain Rose Essential Oils at the company's website and at its headquarters, located in Eugene, Oregon. You may find a selection of these essential oils at a local retailer, as well.

RATINGS AND REVIEWS Customers give Mountain Rose Herbs excellent marks for quality, price, and ease of ordering.

OTHER This company offers a loyalty program and student discounts.

Native American Nutritionals

DESCRIPTION Native American Nutritionals offers an extensive array of single essential oils, blends, and products containing essential oils. This small company focuses on providing organic products.

WHERE TO BUY You can purchase Native American Nutritionals essential oils online and from the company's catalog, which can be ordered online. Some health food stores carry the products, as well.

RATINGS AND REVIEWS Customers give Native American Nutritionals high marks for price, quality, and selection.

OTHER Native American Nutritionals offers a 30-day guarantee on their products.

NOW Foods

DESCRIPTION NOW Foods has been producing natural foods and other supplements since 1948. The company offers a vast array of products, including numerous essential oils, carrier oils, and products containing essential oils.

WHERE TO BUY You can purchase NOW Foods essential oils at some major retailers and online.

RATINGS AND REVIEWS Customers give NOW Foods essential oils good marks for price and quality. These oils are often eclipsed by those offered by smaller companies when compared side by side.

Rocky Mountain Oils

DESCRIPTION Rocky Mountain Oils offers an extensive array of essential oils, blends, and products containing essential oils. Kits and samplers are also available.

WHERE TO BUY You can purchase Rocky Mountain Oils essential oils online and in some retail locations. The company also offers a printed catalog.

RATINGS AND REVIEWS Rocky Mountain Oils has earned excellent marks from customers, particularly as they offer small sampler kits that allow first-time users to try a selection of oils without making a large investment.

OTHER Rocky Mountain Oils has a customer satisfaction guarantee.

STARWEST BOTANICALS

DESCRIPTION Starwest Botanicals offers a wide selection of the most popular essential oils as well as several organic essential oils and essential oil blends. The company has been in business since 1975; today, they are among the largest suppliers of organic herbs and essential oils in the United States.

WHERE TO BUY You can purchase Starwest Botanicals essential oils online and in some health food stores.

RATINGS AND REVIEWS Customers give Starwest Botanicals rave reviews for quality and price.

OTHER Starwest Botanicals offers a 100 percent money-back guarantee in the event a customer is unhappy with an essential oil for any reason.

Young Living

DESCRIPTION Young Living offers several single essential oils, a wide selection of popular blends, and products that contain essential oils.

WHERE TO BUY You can purchase Young Living essential oils online and from independent distributors.

RATINGS AND REVIEWS Some people take exception to the fact that Young Living is a multilevel marketing company; however, the products themselves receive high marks for quality. Customers are particularly satisfied with the company's blended oils.

REFERENCES

Cooksley, Valerie G. *Aromatherapy: A Lifetime Guide to Healing with Essential Oils*. Englewood Cliffs, NJ: Prentice Hall, 1996. Paperback.

Edwards, Victoria H. *The Aromatherapy Companion*. North Adams, MA: Storey Publishing, LLC, 1999.

Eksteins, Angela. "Beware: Adulteration of Essential Oils, Part I." *Natural News*. December 5, 2009. Accessed February 10, 2016. www.naturalnews.com/027661_essential_oils_adulteration.html#.

Falsetto, Sharon. "Scientific Testing of Essential Oils." *Decoded Science*. December 19, 2012. Accessed February 10, 2016. www.decodedscience.com/scientific-testing-of-essential-oils/22544.

Gladstar, Rosemary. *Rosemary Gladstar's Medicinal Herbs: A Beginner's Guide*. North Adams, MA: Storey Publishing, 2012.

Johnson, Dr. Scott A., AMP. *Surviving When Modern Medicine Fails: A Definitive Guide to Essential Oils That Could Save Your Life During a Crisis*. Scott A. Johnson Professional Writing Services, LLC, 2014. Kindle edition.

Keville, Kathi, and Mindy Green. *Aromatherapy: A Complete Guide to the Healing Art*. New York, NY: Crossing Press, 2009.

Lawless, Julia. *The Illustrated Encyclopedia of Essential Oils: The Complete Guide to the Use of Oils in Aromatherapy and Herbalism*. Rockport, MA: Element Books, 1995.

Meamarbashi, Abbas, and Ali Rajabi. "The Effects of Peppermint on Exercise Performance." U.S. National Library of Medicine, National Institutes of Health. March 21, 2013. Accessed February 12, 2016. www.ncbi.nlm.nih.gov/pmc/articles/PMC3607906/.

White, Gregory L. *Essential Oils and Aromatherapy: How to Use Essential Oils for Beauty, Health, and Spirituality.* White Willow Books, 2013.

Wildwood, Chrissie. *The Encyclopedia of Aromatherapy.* Rochester, VT: Healing Arts Press, 1996.

Worwood, Valerie Ann. *The Complete Book of Essential Oils and Aromatherapy.* Novato, CA: New World Library, 1991.

Worwood, Valerie Ann. *The Fragrant Mind: Aromatherapy for Personality, Mind, Mood and Emotion.* Novato, CA: New World Library, 1996.

INDEX OF AILMENTS AND REMEDIES

C

F

H

M

N

O

P

R

S

T

V

W

Y

INDEX OF ESSENTIAL OILS

R

S

T

V

Y

INDEX

ABOUT THE AUTHOR

ANNE KENNEDY began her lifelong study of herbs and plants as a child in Montana's Bitterroot Valley, starting with an interest in Native American herbal remedies. Today she is a writer who specializes in a wide variety of natural health, gardening, and sustainability topics. She has written several books on essential oils and herbal medicine, including *Essential Oils Natural Remedies* and *Essential Oils for Beginners*. Self-sufficiency, an active outdoor lifestyle, and a strong focus on the interconnectedness of body, mind, and spirit serve as her inspiration and cornerstone for healthy living. Anne lives and works from her home on a small organic farm in the mountains of West Virginia. Her favorite essential oil is frankincense.